Test Positive

Test Positive

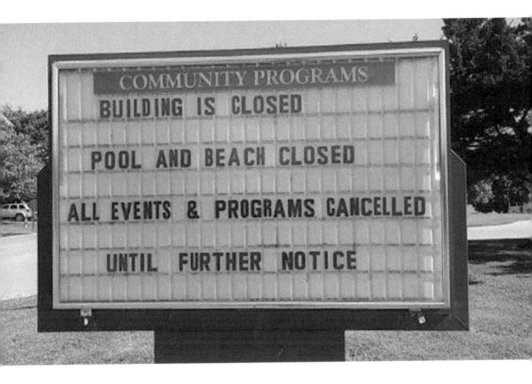

Surviving COVID-19 in
the Reign of Trump

Gerard Plecki, Ph. D.

MILL CITY PRESS

Mill City Press, Inc.
2301 Lucien Way #415
Maitland, FL 32751
407.339.4217
www.millcitypress.net

Library of Congress Control Number: 2021901440

Paperback ISBN-13: 978-1-6322-1368-6
Hardcover ISBN-13: 978-1-6322-1369-3

Ebook ISBN-13: 978-1-6322-1370-9

Table of Contents

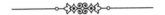

Preface

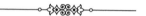

I am not a scientist, a doctor, a politician, a talk-show host, a reporter, or a tele-evangelist. I am an average, sixty-nine-year old male, six foot one inches tall. I weighed one hundred and eighty-five pounds prior to my two-month struggle for survival. Because of my age and a history of underlying medical conditions, when I tested positive to COVID-19, I fell in the category of those most susceptible to dying from the disease.

When I became aware that I was sick, I was aghast to learn that there were no indices available to tell me what I should expect to encounter each day. There were no data on what symptoms I would encounter, how long each symptom would last, how to rank the severity of my systems, or how much time it would take me to recover. I had assumed that because I lived in the most technologically and medically advanced nation in the world, I would be able to examine the information that we had accumulated in a federal database. I thought I would be able to determine where I fell on a continuum scaled from "you will probably live" to "make sure your affairs are in order."

I discovered to my dismay that my assumption was completely and totally inaccurate. There was no specific information to be found online. Doctors did not know of any "typical" progression of the disease. No data was available from the Center for Disease Control and Prevention, which was an organization I was confident would have organized data based on hundreds of thousands of case reports. No federal agency was forthcoming with information that I knew would be valuable to anyone who had been infected with the Coronavirus. The President of the United States assured us that our symptoms would be no more severe than what we would experience if we had caught a common cold.

I decided that if I survived COVID-19, I would provide a detailed account of what I experienced during my two months-plus of illness. My hope was that if anyone fighting the disease had a blueprint for what they might reasonably expect to encounter as they fought COVID-19, their levels of fear and anxiety would be reduced.

Left to my own devices, when I learned that no vaccine or medical therapy was effective and efficacious in fighting the disease, I developed a holistic approach for attacking the Coronavirus. I cannot make an authoritative or quantifiable claim that the regimen I followed helped me defeat COVID-19. My survival might have been due to the size of Coronavirus dosage that I received, to the amount of time I was exposed to the Coronavirus, to the normal functioning of my immune system, to prayer, or to plain, dumb luck. I can produce only anecdotal evidence to bolster my hope that what worked for me might work for anyone else who tests positive for COVID-19. Although I cannot state with absolute certainty that my actions saved my life, I believe that to be the case. I also believe that with prayer, with an ironclad resolution to survive, and armed with a protocol similar to the one I describe in this book, anyone who tests positive for Coronavirus infection will have a greater chance of surviving the disease.

I also resolved not to add misinformation about COVID-19 causes and "remedies" to the mountains of unsubstantiated assertions proposed by certain politicians whose actions are geared toward augmenting their re-election chances, not toward helping the average American survive this horribly-infectious and deadly pandemic. I have been as objective as possible about the nature and extent of my illness, and about the historical context within which it occurred, because offering a jeremiad would do no one any good.

As I wrestled with COVID-19, I was consistently astounded by the lack of authoritative information about what happens hour to hour, day to day, and week to week to anyone fighting this virus. As a patient, I felt an obligation to inform others of the challenges they can reasonably expect to encounter when locking horns with the Coronavirus. As a historian, I was compelled to examine the politics of the pandemic, as its conceptualization evolved from a "like a cold" prognosis in January and February to an uncontrolled pandemic in July 2020.

For months we had been told tacit and outright lies by an ego-driven politician who is content to talk a big game but do nothing to stop the spread of the Coronavirus. I felt it important to communicate the danger we face as a nation when those political deceptions and omissions are exacerbated and excused by provocative, right-wing media outlets.

When I finished writing this book, nearly five million Americans had tested positive to COVID-19. Four percent of those people have died needlessly. A million other people suffered through the disease as I did, and narrowly escaped death. It is the legacy bequeathed to us by President Donald J. Trump.

We cannot pretend that the palliations and denials that were thrust upon us from January to March 2020 did not occur. We were given assurances that the Coronavirus posed no threat to our lives. Months later, when each claim proved to be untrue, politicians denied making those statements. Federal action was required to save our lives, and though none took place, we were later asked to believe that our government had acted wisely and responsibly. Bewildered by those prevarications, we wondered if anyone in our government cared if we lived or died. Nursing home patients, health care providers, emergency responders, members of ethnic and disadvantaged communities, employees at meat-packing facilities, the elderly, the incarcerated, and the infirmed soon learned the disheartening answer to that question.

This book is humbly dedicated to everyone who has struggled with a COVID-19 infection. Your fight has been a valiant one, and it has not gone unnoticed. To that end, I wish all those whose lives have been threatened by COVID-19 my sincerest hopes and prayers for survival, and Godspeed in recovery. In the words of the rock group The Call, "Here's to you my loves, with blessings from Above, let the day begin." Let us hope that the day will be begin on November 3, when a responsible person takes the Oath of Office and assumes the leadership of our country.

Chapter One

武汉

Ground Zero

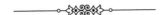

If we were asked to speculate on what passes for daily existence in Central China, many of us would conjure a drab, colorless landscape, with caves and hovels as homes for pitiful residents. Those forlorn inhabitants would be cursed to eke out joyless lives in some backwater village where the buses do not run, located at the intersection of You're Screwed Avenue and Hell on Earth Highway. They would carry home a day's supply of potable water and meager foodstuffs in rickshaws that were generations old. If parents were lucky enough to have jobs working in a rice paddy in the rain for sixteen hours a day, then those earnings could be used to feed their one and only son, who has trudged the three miles home from pseudo-military school. After having his dinner, he would walk to the local dungeon where he would begin his ten-hour shift sewing shoes or shirts for eight yen a day.

His dinner might have consisted of some mammal that Noah wanted to leave behind when he gathered his troops two by two, but somehow the devilish creature had found its way to the rafters of his Ark. Millenia later, our Central China family members would feast on the tasty treat that they had purchased at, bartered for, or stolen from a rabid garden of earthly delights called a wet market.

Looking out through a glassless window frame from the front of a two-room shack called home, an unlucky resident would see row after row of burning trashcans used to counter the chill of wintry nights. The skyline, if it could be called that, would resemble barrios dug into the hillside suburbs of Rio de Janeiro. A climb to the top of a hill would reveal nothing more than a desolate, barren landscape, unencumbered by trees, parks, high-rises, or by any manmade structure that could testify that this was indeed the twenty-first century.

Life in Wuhan City in Central China, however, is quite different from any stereotype we would imagine. As the capital of China's Hubei Province, it boasts a population of eleven million, and as such, it has the ninth highest population of all China cities. It is a manufacturing and industrial hub. Its edifices include the fifteen hundred-foot tall Wuhan Center, the Yellow Crane Tower, the Minsheng Bank Building, and the Wuhan World Trade Center. Other soon-to-be-completed skyscrapers will include the Phoenix Towers and the Wuhan Greenland Center, both of which will rival Dubai's Burj Khalifa in height.

In the past few decades, Wuhan has been the subject of several international news stories. In 2000, for example, a Wuhan Airlines flight encountered a thunderstorm and crashed, killing everyone on board and a dozen people residing near the Han River. In 2008 the United States opened its consulate for Central China in Wuhan. In 2016, heavy rainfall caused the Han to overflow, resulting in many deaths and forcing the relocation of one hundred thousand residents. In October 2019, Wuhan hosted the Seventh International CISM Military World Games.

Wuhan has more colleges and universities than any other China city. With so much focus on higher education, one could reasonably expect to find a large scientific and technological presence within the confines of the city, and one would not be disappointed. Nearly a half million researchers and consultants are employed at more than two thousand Wuhan facilities.

Perhaps less admirably, such widespread interest in science and technology has allowed Wuhan to become the number one source of synthetic opioids in the world. Drug cartels love the cheap prices of the base chemicals used in a product sold to many interested parties in the United States.

Worse though is the fact that in 2015, the Wuhan Institute of Virology, located in the city's Jiangxia District, began to operate the country's first

Level Four biological research laboratory. Though the exact scope, purpose, and tenor of research conducted at that facility has never been made public, it is safe to assume that not all experiments conducted at Level Four were undertaken for humanitarian purposes. In fact, Biosafety Level 4 labs are built to develop and study viruses like Ebola which can be weaponized to cause hemorrhagic fever.

According to the Federation of American Scientists, not many of these BSL-4 labs exist in the world. Most of them are located in the USA, and they can be found at two Center of Disease Control and Prevention labs in Atlanta and in Fort Collins, Colorado; at the Center for Biodefense and Emerging Infectious Diseases at the University of Texas in Galveston; at the Center for Biotechnology and Drug Design at Georgia State University in Atlanta; at the Southwest Foundation for Biomedical Research in San Antonio, and at the Rocky Mountain Laboratories Integrated Research Facilities in Hamilton, Montana. The Montana site is run by the National Institute of Health, which should not be confused with the National Institute of Allergy and Infectious Diseases, the organization headed since 1984 by Dr. Anthony Fauci.

Our facilities share the same spectrum of interests with the Wuhan Institute of Virology. As parts of their mission statements, these august institutions study the development of biological and chemical weaponry, the storage of lethal and nonlethal chemical and biological weapons, delivery systems for that weaponry, registration of and education about those weapons, and the investigation and development of threat agents. No one running these BSL-4 labs seems interested in curing the common cold or improving the general lot of mankind. The plain fact is that the enterprises in these establishments could be characterized as more sinister than benevolent in nature. On the positive side, if we are bombarded with pathogens from distant shores of the Milky Way Galaxy, a BSL-4 laboratory is exactly what we need to study the origin of those species.

Although I believe in coincidence as much as the next person, it may not be reasonable to assume that the connection between a BSL-4 lab experimenting on highly infectious pathogens, and the presence of one such pathogen in a so-called "wet market" is purely coincidental. Many of the employees of said lab routinely shop for bargain-priced entrees in that market, buying things that no one in their right mind in our culture would consider ingesting.

For such a coincidence to occur, one would have to ignore three facts: according to the World Health Organization, the Institute has had a "history of studying coronavirus in bats;" China has a "lax safety record in its labs;" and the Virology lab is located in close proximity "to where some of the infections were first diagnosed."[1]

Officials at the Wuhan Institute of Virology and state-controlled media spokespersons have denied no fewer than a hundred times that the Coronavirus was made in a lab. Such statements do not address a more important question: how did the virus that was being studied in the lab make its way to the wet market? Conceding that the virus was not man-made, if there is a connection between the virus studied in that BSL-4 lab and the presence of the same virus in horseshoe bats sold at the wet market—a connection which the Institute has also vigorously denied—then either a bat escaped from Level 4 containment and found its way to the wet market, or the virus was transmitted by an infected, perhaps asymptomatic employee. Since a bat is probably too large of a creature to escape easily from BSL-4 containment, the second scenario seems more likely.

The infected Institute employee would have spread the Coronavirus to everyone he encountered as he meandered from aisle to aisle at the wet market, in the same manner and with the same heightened degree of interest that we would display when comparing brands of corn flakes at the Piggly-Wiggly. Unsuspecting shoppers would have brought the virus home with them along with their fresh fruits, vegetables, and any mammals they may have purchased, the same way Jacksonville beachgoers brought home a tan and the Coronavirus after their Memorial Day and Fourth of July outings.

The Virology Institute had assembled a good-sized collection of horseshoe bats as test subjects. The immune system of bats allows the animal to carry without harm to itself a hundred different diseases, any one of which would sicken or kill us. All sorts of viruses reside in the "ecological reservoir" of a bat's immune system. The Novel Coronavirus, technically called SARS-CoV-2, was one such pathogen hosted by the horseshoe bat. Perhaps an Institute employee whose job it was to dissect the bat touched its blood and its other bodily fluids, and in doing so, the terrain where the Coronavirus lived was exposed. Perhaps that person was a bit too "lax" when it was time to decontaminate the massive amount of personal protective equipment that everyone at Level 4 wore, before the worker cleared the airlocks and entered the world at large. Perhaps that person's PPE was of the same poor quality as the PPE the federal government sent to nursing homes in June 2020. If this person contracted the Coronavirus at his or her place of employment, a random cough, a shout, or a sneeze at the wet market could have easily started the ball rolling in Wuhan City.

It is also a fact that the horseshoe bats sold at the wet market carried the virus. Hundreds of bats were sold each day the wet market was open; it was a practice that had gone on for decades. Oddly enough, it was not until the Wuhan Institute of Virology became fully operational and started dissecting more bats than Nolan Ryan had faced in his entire career that the Wuhan City outbreak began.

To suppose that this virus initiated and activated itself by happenstance at the wet market does not explain how the Coronavirus jumped the species barrier between animal and human. The swine flu was deadly because it combined avian flu with an additional oomph it received from the pig's own DNA. No two animals combined viruses at the wet market, but that was one of the specific, experimental processes being studied at Wuhan City's Institute of Virology's BSL-4 laboratory.

A simpler way to consider the problem is to start with the assumption that patient zero in this quagmire might have been an Institute employee or a random test subject who, through either intent and purpose or simple carelessness, became infected with the virus and left the facility. Once outside the lab's hermetically sealed doors, that person may or may not have visited the wet market. Whether he or she went shopping or stopped at the Yida Football Music Bar for a Tsingtao or visited Mansion KTV for a few rounds of karaoke, anyone who might have had the simple and colossal misfortune of being at the wrong place at the wrong time would have become infected.

It is also possible that patient zero might have touched or breathed upon other animate or inanimate objects before returning home for dinner. For example, if contact of any sort had been made with a horseshoe bat, then that specific strain of SARS-CoV-2 could have found its way into the bat's "reservoir." If contact had made with any food item in the market-place, transmission could have occurred when that food was prepared and consumed. Whether a randomly infected bat bought at the wet market had been sliced, diced, or fricasseed, transmission would have followed as surely as night follows day.

At a White House Coronavirus Task Force briefing on April 22, 2020, a reporter asked Dr. Fauci if the virus could find a way to travel from pet to humans, or from humans to pets. Dr. Fauci stated that the virus can affect multiple species, and that anything is possible, but "there is no evidence that we've see, from an epidemiological standpoint, that pets can be transmitters within the household."

Since Dr. Fauci's response addressed the unlikelihood of the virus jumping species barriers, President Trump, in his full-on "Aren't I clever?" mode, asked Dr. Fauci how a lion in the zoo got infected. Dr. Fauci's reply was particularly relevant to the question of how transmission from Patient Zero might have occurred in Wuhan City. It also clarified the mechanics of cross-species transmission of the zoonotic disease commonly known as COVID-19. He stated, "I don't know, Mr. President, but I would imagine that one of the zookeepers probably had an asymptomatic infection, took care of the animals, gave them some food, touched them, whatever, that's how he got it."

In the 2013 Marc Forster film World War Z, the virologist Dr. Fassbach (Eyles Gabel), who had been tasked with finding a vaccine for the zombie virus, told UN investigator Gerry Lane (Brad Pitt) that "Once we find its origin we can develop a vaccine." After traveling to South Korea and Israel, Lane reached the conclusion that it will be impossible to find the source.

The true cause of the Wuhan outbreak may forever remain a riddle, wrapped in a mystery, inside an enigma. We certainly cannot accept at face value the multitude of various disclaimers issued by Yuan Zhiming, the Director of the Institute, and by government spokespersons. What we can conclude is that there could be a high positive correlation between pathogen work at China's only BSL-4 laboratory with a record of lax safety protocols, and the manifestation of said pathogen in a marketplace in close proximity to that lab.

It would make sense that Chinese officials would feel comfortable propagating a cover story which sourced the outbreak to horseshoe bats sold at the wet market. By admitting to the popularity of a sensational practice—eating bats—which the rest of the civilized world would view as unseemly, they would steer attention away from a more dangerous truth, that their own lax BSL-4 safety protocols had permitted a virus to escape and endanger anyone with whom it came into contact.

Throughout the lockdown of Wuhan City, Zhiming's labs remained open for business, plugging away at its daily, ho-hum routine of finding new and more efficient ways to threaten the existence of every man, woman, child, and animal in the world. It is not surprising that on February 7, when most of the city's lockdown restrictions were lifted, Yuan Zhiming, impervious and ostensibly blameless for the outbreak, conducted a soiree celebrating the Grand Re-Opening of Wuhan City.

At 1a.m. on April 8, the Institute hosted the best damned laser-light show ever witnessed by the assembled and bedazzled multitude. Heavy appetizers were not be provided for the throngs by concessioners of the Huanan Seafood Wholesale Market of Wuhan. Like the barndoors that were closed after the proverbial horses had escaped, the wet market was closed on January 1, 2020, to protect the health and welfare of the rich or poor, employed or unemployable, healthy or already-sick residents of Wuhan City. Nearly four thousand persons could not attend. They had a previous date with destiny, involving six feet of bulldozed earth in a mass gravesite in Hubei Province.

The accuracy of that figure was not established until nine days after the light show, when government officials announced that the Wuhan death toll was fifty-percent higher than anticipated. The updated figure showed that three thousand, eight hundred and sixty-nine residents had succumbed to the disease. It was the same type of "miscalculation" that characterized our federal government's report on the number of deaths in our nursing homes, which was made public in the second week of June 2020.

The temporary shuttering of the Wuhan City wet market did little to slow the avalanche of disease and death which would befall one hundred and eighty-four nations. Five weeks after the closing of the that auspicious market, on February 6, the Chinese death toll was reported to have risen to seven hundred and twenty-two. On that date, the first United States of America citizen died from the Novel Coronavirus. Reuters stated the person was a sixty-year-old man; the New York Times thought the person was a woman with underlying medical problems. Either way, the person had been in quarantine in a Wuhan medical staging area for a month.

Those medical staging areas did not resemble any hospital that Americans had ever seen. A better descriptor of those facilities would be "death warehouses." Once quarantined in one of those locations, it was first come, first served; early arrivals would be given beds, later ones would sit on plastic chairs. Whether one was stationed in a bed or chair, the game plan was the same: if one survived, it was by luck of the draw. There were no ventilators to help them breathe. Lack of food did not matter much to patients in their final days; Coronavirus victims have little appetite. It was by far a grimmer situation than one would care to imagine possible in the twenty-first century.

On our soil, the first two death from Coronavirus occurred in Santa Clara County, California, on February 6 and February 17. In the state of Washington on February 29, the death of a man in his fifties was attributed to the Novel Coronavirus. The first death from the Coronavirus in South Korea occurred on February 20. If our country and South Korea had responded in similar fashions, then after adjusting for the difference in population size, the death toll should have been similar. By mid-May though, two hundred and sixty-four people in South Korea had died, compared to an extraordinarily and obscenely disproportionate eighty thousand Americans who died from COVID-19 in the United States.

One might reasonably wonder what our federal government was doing to protect its citizens during this crucial, two-month period from mid-February to mid-April. We might wonder what would have been the result if our government had acted as early and efficiently as South Korea's government and had similar programs of social distancing mitigation, contact tracing, surveillance tracing, and most importantly, uniform and widespread testing. On April 16, The Hill.com reported that if we had put social distancing measures in place by March 2, the percent of U.S. deaths due to COVID-19 would have decreased by ninety percent; if they had been in place by March 9, the number of American deaths would have decreased by sixty percent.[2]

Tragically, neither of those timelines were met. Instead, on January 22, when four hundred and forty cases and seventeen deaths from Novel Coronavirus had occurred in China, President Trump stated, "We have it totally under control...it's going to be just fine." He made this unsubstantiated prediction on the day after the first U.S. case was diagnosed in Washington State, which was more than a month after the first case of COVID-19-was diagnosed in Chicago, on January 24. On February 24, President Trump tweeted "The Coronavirus is very much under control in the USA" and that the "Stock Market (is) starting to look very good to me!" On February 27 he declared "It's going to disappear. One day, it's like a miracle, it will disappear." During these two months, Trump maintained that the virus was like a common cold or a flu which "goes away in April with the heat."

Although this "flu" did not go away in April, President Trump stood by the accuracy of his diagnosis. During a White House Coronavirus Task Force briefing on April 23 he poignantly illustrated his belief in the miraculous way the virus would disappear. When a Department of Homeland Security administrator William Bryan stated that the virus did not do well when conditions of high temperature and sunlight prevailed, our President jumped to the next illogical conclusion, because this was exactly the "evidence" he needed, the magic bullet which supported his belief in the Miracle of the Disappearing Coronavirus. Stating that since summer was almost here, all the American public needed to do was to wait a little bit longer. The problem—which a dyspeptic Trump has labelled The China Virus, The Plague, The Unseen Enemy, The Curse, and the Kung Flu—would certainly disappear.

He was certain that Florida, with its heat and humidity, could soon open its beaches, and crowds could gather to watch the Thunderbirds and Blue Angels airshows, which he believed would be a grand way to celebrate the Re-Opening of the Country. The Wuhan Lightshow would pale when compared to the festivities Las Vegas offered when the MGM Hotel Resort opened for business on June 4. The mall in downtown Las Vegas had its own considerable lightshow which could be easily adapted to entertain all Coronavirus-carrying patrons spending their twelve-hundred-dollar Trump check at the first vacant roulette wheel or slot machine they spotted.

In an astonishing exchange during this same briefing, Mr. Bryan stated the Coronavirus died quickly in lab experiments when it was exposed to ultraviolet light and isopropyl alcohol. Upon hearing this news, President Trump's excitement was visceral. In front of the White House Press and millions of Americans watching the Task Force briefing, President Trump asked if there was any way to inject a disinfectant into the body, or to insert an ultraviolet light source to "clean out" the lungs. His specific words regarding the healing power of Lysol were, "And then I see the disinfectant where it knocks it out in a minute—one minute—and is there a way we can do something like that by injection inside, or almost a cleaning? Because you see it gets in the lungs and it does a tremendous number on the lungs, so it would be interesting to check that." Our Commander in Chief was unaware that disinfectants kill humans dumb enough to swallow or inject themselves with those chemicals. He was unaware that several hundred Iranians had died from drinking isopropyl.

It was clear that President Trump lacked a high schooler's understanding that the human body does not react well when exposed to a significant amount of ultraviolet radiation.

He was moderately disappointed in the reply he received from one of his Task Force scientists, Dr. Deborah Brix, when he hypothesized, "Supposing we hit the body with a tremendous, whether it's ultraviolet or just very powerful light, supposing you brought the light inside the body, either through the skin or some other way" to kill the cursed Coronavirus. She suppressed the grimace which was her first reaction to his question and answered tactfully, "Not as a treatment."

It did not require telepathic powers to read Trump's mind at that moment. From his facial expression and harried gestures, it was clear he was thinking, "I've got to get some mileage out of this, it's so close, the problem is almost solved, and once I solve it using my good old common sense and my remarkable powers of deduction, everyone will call me The Miracle Worker." His statements about the efficacy of ultraviolet light as a therapeutic measure resulted in the average American receiving several dozen spam emails offering cheap prices on "Blue Light Blocking Sunglasses." The busines plan was that for the right price, anyone intent on blasting themselves with ultraviolet radiation would probably want to protect their retinas.

Solar energy proponents understand that the presence of bright, sunny days in April is intermittent at best; the glass-half-full side of that equation meant to President Trump that April showers would certainly add enough humidity to the air to defeat the Unseen Enemy. On that same date of April 23, twenty-six thousand, one hundred and forty residents of Orleans and Jefferson Parishes in Louisiana rightfully took issue with Trump's logic. High humidity did not save them from testing positive. Seven thousand cases owned by residents of New Orleans, resulted in more than sixteen hundred deaths.

To place President Trump's statements in January and February 2020 within a proper context, we must remember that President Trump had been alerted to the threat of a pandemic in November and December 2019. Those warnings, coming from his intelligence committees, were completely ignored. On January 29, when the first two Coronavirus cases were reported in Lombardi, Italy, White House advisor Peter Navarro sent President Trump a memo explaining why the Novel Coronavirus outbreak in China posed a serious threat to the safety of our citizens. The memo spurred President Trump to ban flights from China; nevertheless, he permitted an estimated forty thousand Chinese citizens to enter the USA after the "ban" was imposed. It was an allowance which proved to be irrecoverable. The President took no action at that time to prohibit travel from Italy into the United States. The main port of entry from Italy and from most of Europe was New York's JFK International Airport. We will never know how many New Yorker's lives would have been spared if President Trump had provided more than a knee-jerk rejection of Navarro's admonition.

On February 23, Navarro rang another alarm, repeating his warning in sterner terms. He began his memo to the President by stating a "full-blown COVID-19 pandemic could infect as many as 100 million Americans and kill as many as 1.2 million." Navarro wrote that the Coronavirus constituted a "crisis that could inflict trillions of dollars in economic damage and take millions of lives."[3] His words fell on deaf ears.

While our President scoffed at the mere mention of "pandemic," while he did nothing when common sense and a survival instinct should have motivated him to take steps necessary to save the lives of Americans, China recognized the severity of the situation it had created and acted quickly to curtail the death of its citizens. The China outbreak peaked on February 16, with nineteen thousand, four hundred and fifty-seven cases reported. One week later, that number dropped to a mere two-hundred and fourteen cases. The virtual elimination of new cases was the result of widescale testing, strict quarantine measures, and the cessation of train travel to and from all major Chinese population centers, including Hong Kong. China devised and implemented a national emergency plan to deal with the crisis; although the measures taken were draconian in nature and subjected the population to major inconveniences for a short period of time, the outbreak was contained and millions of lives were spared.

Lest China's actions sound altruistic, we should remember that its concern about the Coronavirus outbreak ended at its borders. China did not care about what happened to the rest of the world. A Chinese statement of responsibility followed by an action plan to stop the virus from spreading to other nations would have been appreciated by everyone else populating Planet Earth. But such an acknowledgement was not forthcoming. No steps were taken to stop Coronavirus carriers from leaving the country. The flow of Coronavirus carriers to every country, from Afghanistan to Zimbabwe, was unchecked. Planes, trains, and boatloads of Chinese citizens, relatives, and visitors to China departed in an unabated fashion. Humans became the rats of the Black Plague; the Coronavirus was the flea that each rat carried.

Like many European cities, Italy relied on a large Chinese work force to meet its need for employees in manufacturing and light industry jobs. Each flight from Beijing, Shanghai, Hong Kong, and Guangzhou to Milan, Rome, Venice, Bologna, and Naples brought three hundred more employees, supervisors, friends, and relatives from the Mainland. Many of them were either asymptomatic or symptomatic carriers of the Coronavirus. Although Italy closed the city of Lombardi, which was its ground zero, and eventually banned all flights from China, the damage had already been done.

On February 23, seventy-one cases were reported nationwide. One month later, the daily number of new cases had reached six thousand. For the next three weeks, between four thousand and seven thousand new cases were reported each day. One month after that, the country reported a minimum of four thousand new cases per day. Two months later, the number of deaths in Italy had reached twenty-six thousand, three hundred and eight-four, and had claimed the lives of thirteen thousand, one hundred and six residents of Lombardi. This pattern of transmission and incubation, followed a few weeks later by major outbreaks, was repeated in Spain, in other European countries, and in the UK.

One would assume that after watching these scenarios unfold in Europe and comparing them to how China handled its crisis, our federal government officials would reach an obvious conclusion. Since the China model worked and the European model failed miserably to limit the spread of the disease, our country should immediately take whatever steps necessary to institute a well-considered, cogent, unilateral, national emergency plan to limit the spread of Coronavirus in this country. Mitigation by social distancing, testing, and mask wearing would later come into play, but in the final week of February, steps should have been taken to outline how to effectuate quarantine measures and actualize containment plans.

To ignore the seriousness of the threat constituted criminal negligence. Even though it was certain that most Americans would not have liked the plan, and consequently political futures would be at risk, steps should have been taken to protect the Homeland. If banning flights from China had actually prevented Coronavirus carriers from entering the country from China, it would have been a step in the right direction, but because the ban was ineffective at its initial, crucial stages, lives were lost. A ban on China flights was not a cure all, despite how eagerly our President publicized each singular action, event, or discovery as The Solution to the Pandemic. A multi-faceted plan of attack was desperately needed, and as February approached its end, the United States of America lacked any such strategy.

On February 24, President Trump declared "We are in contact with everyone and all relevant countries. CDC & World Health have been working hard and very smart." Two months later he castigated the W.H.O. and threatened to cut off all USA funding for that organization.

He tweeted on February 25, "U.S. acted on the Coronavirus very, very quickly." On February 26, he told reports at the James S. Brady Press Briefing Room "the number one priority from our standpoint is the health and safety of the American people. And that's the way I viewed it when I made that decision. Because of all we've done, the risk to the American people remains very low. The United States is now—we're rated number one. We're rated number one for being prepared."

The President had just returned from a fact-finding mission to India and bragged about the success of the trip. India was about to experience its own Coronavirus problems, coming on the heels of its armed border conflicts with its neighboring nuclear power, China. After reporters patiently listened to Trump complimenting himself and Prime Minister Modi, claiming that Modi would send "billions and billions of dollars now to the United States"—a claim that never actualized— reporters turned questions back to the elephant in the room, the worldwide pandemic. President Trump ingenuously declared "Well, I don't think it's inevitable...whatever happens, we're totally prepared."

When asked "as the virus spreads in Italy and South Korea, are you planning on adding those countries to the list?" Trump abdicated responsibility by stating, "Well, just so you understand—you know, I'm the President of the United States. I'm not the President of other countries. I don't think it's right to impose our self on others." Trump was not asked if he was going to impose his will on other countries, he was directly asked what *he* is going to do to stop the Coronavirus from spreading to the USA from those countries. It is important to note that this pattern of dancing around questions he *does not* like and giving an irrelevant answer that he *does* like would be repeated endlessly. The Brady Room became his Romper Room.

One reporter who would not be sidetracked from the obvious asked two questions that would be considered "leading" in any court of law: "Mr. President, have you made any plans that would involve quarantined cities, like we saw in China? And what would have to happen for you to take a step like that?" The only way the reporter's intent could have been more obvious is if he held a sign, begging Trump to "please do something that works like it did in China, not something that doesn't work like it didn't work in Italy!" Demonstrating his consistent willingness to obfuscate, which has been and continues to be his default position, President Trump ranted with bald-faced effrontery, "We do have plans of a much—on a much larger scale, should we need that. We're working with states, we're working with virtually every state. And we do have plans on a larger scale if we need it. We don't think we're going to need it, but, you know, you always have to be prepared."

The sad truth is that there was absolutely no preparation underway, no federal plan to save lives, no willingness to work with states. In fact, the President displayed an easily discernible predilection toward making things more difficult for blue states to handle the developing crisis. The suggestion that there was a grand scheme, a secret plan in place, one so well-conceived that it would embrace any challenge and quickly resolve any developing complexity was at best a brazen notion, at worst a conscious deception, a replacement of facts with idle speculation and pie-in-the-sky conjecture.

His inclusion of the disclaimer "if we need it" foisted upon an uninformed American public his deluded notion that there was no cause for alarm. We were to believe that his genius for governing the country would make the Coronavirus pandemic disappear, as though it was a gnat one could swat away with a flick of the wrist. In later Task Force briefings, the President would contradict or explain away such truly bogus statements. He used doublespeak to prove he had acted correctly right down the line. When he was called on the carpet for making the reductive "if we need it" aphorism, he denied making the statement. In doing so, he accomplished the neat, twofold task of abrogating responsibility and becoming his own Judas Iscariot.

Before Mission Control ignited the Saturn V rocket that launched Apollo 11 to the moon, the three astronauts completed a rigorous check list. Each item on the list proved to be "nominal, A-OK." In his each of his Task Force briefings and press conferences, President Trump followed NASA protocol and told the country that everything is "A-OK." When he was asked during the February 26 briefing about the country's supply of face coverings and personal protective equipment, he provided yet another example of his eagerness to fiddle while Rome burned. He stated, "We've ordered a lot of it just in case we need it. We may not need it; you understand that. But in case—we're looking at worst-case scenario. We're going to be set very quickly." Naturally, every word in his reply was suspect. No abundance of masks was on hand; "a lot of it" had not been ordered; and as the "worst-case scenario" knocked at our door, President Trump ensconced himself in the role of the ever courteous, always helpful valet, the obsequious "cheerleader," the glad-handing politician who, as Commander in Chief, stated as fact what he thought we wanted to hear.

We deserve and we must demand so much more than that from our nation's leader, in times of crisis and in times of celebration. If we are told a plan is in place, then a plan should exist, and we should be informed of what that plan involves and what sacrifices it requires from us. It is unconscionable that with so many lives at stake, Task Force briefings became political rallies, where somber reporters were humiliated each day for asking tough questions, where the ambience of the Briefing reeked with the same desultory smugness and lying condescension that we last witnessed in the Nixon-Agnew era. Because impeachment was a badge of honor for President Trump, it is expecting too much to think he might have learned something about fair play from that unpleasantness. But no lesson was learned; the process was empowering for him because it was a "fake impeachment." Anyone else would have thought to clean up his or her act, but not our President. Instead, his lies and deflections during the pandemic provided us with a reanimated General James Mattoon Scott, a strutting egoist with a Napoleonic power complex, a caricature who lacked Scott's tempered eloquence, his emotionless intelligence, and his mistrust of Russians.

Instead, after twice calling Speaker Nancy Pelosi incompetent, a piqued President said that Cryin' Chuck Schumer "shouldn't be making statements like that, because it's so bad for the country." He scolded Schumer, saying "we should be working together," thereby demonstrating his own clinical inability to practice what he preaches. If President Trump wished to "work together" to solve a problem which was either "very little" or "could be very big"—depending on from which side of his mouth he was speaking—he would stop the name-calling and blue-baiting that resounded throughout his campaign for election, throughout his tenure in office, and in each of his Task Force briefings.

After explaining that he had sued the editor of <u>The New York Times</u> for writing an op-ed piece with which disagreed, he boasted "we're testing everybody that we need to test, and we're finding very little problem, very little problem." No criterion for "need" was established, and no delineation of what "everybody" meant was produced. The testing timeframe was nonspecific, and the location where this alleged testing would occur was, at best guess, where the sun does not shine.

It was at this briefing that Dr. Tony Fauci introduced himself as Director of the National Institute of Allergy and Infectious Diseases. He gave what he called "a very quick update on the countermeasure development in the form of vaccines and therapeutics." In less than two minutes he provided the American public with a concise explanation of what steps were required to test various therapeutic agents and to produce a vaccine. Regarding therapeutics, he explained that the anti-viral drugs such as remdesivir would be subjected to standard clinical trials before their efficacy and safety could be evaluated. About a vaccine, he stated that "if this virus—which we have every reason to believe it is quite conceivable that it will happen—will go beyond just a season and come back and recycle next year—if that's the case, we hope to have a vaccine."

In an often repeated and tragically pathetic cycle, President Trump attempted with little success to reject or walk back such scientific conclusions as Dr. Fauci's. By rejecting facts he did not like about the Coronavirus pandemic, President Trump demonstrated a pathological drive to muddy the waters, to offer his "instinctive," Know-Nothing beliefs as though he was the adept game show host who knew what was hidden behind Door Number Two. To place this in another context—an equally unfortunate one for the American public—there was never a choice for us between the lady or the tiger. As days and weeks moved along and the numbers of cases and deaths rose, the option President Trump offered was the tiger, or the tiger.

The outbreak in a nursing home in Kirkland, Washington did nothing to spur President Trump into action. The Life Care Center long-term nursing facility was home to one hundred and twenty residents. The first patient from the Center suffering from undiagnosed COVID-19 symptoms was hospitalized on February 19. In the next two weeks, twenty-six of its residents died, and many of the deaths occurred surprising quickly. Within hours of showing no symptoms of COVID-19, a patient would be hospitalized and die.

The progression of the disease turned on a dime. This fact differentiated it from any typical flu timeframe, and for these reasons, the

Coronavirus should have raised a red flag at the highest level of our Federal Government. It did not. When the individuals who were the first responders to Life Care Center 911 calls became ill and died shortly thereafter, the red flag had become an alarm bell screaming for federal attention. Those sirens went unheard by the Trump administration.

Washington's Governor Jay Inslee understood that this disease posed a real threat to his constituents and he ordered nursing facilities first to curtail visiting hours, then to prohibit visitors at any affected facility. Unlike President Trump, who regarded nursing home residents as the 2020 equivalent of Hunter Thompson's The Doomed, Governor Inslee recognized two irrefutable facts: that he must do what he could to save the lives of nursing home residents, and that nursing homes did not exist in a vacuum. Employees were members of a larger community, and if they were infected and not quarantined, they would transmit the Coronavirus to whomever they contacted.

Officials in several suburbs of Seattle recognized that a very real threat of community transmission existed. When the relative of a Bothell High School employee tested positive, that school was closed. Others followed suit.

True to his myopic nature, though, President Trump could not recognize this microcosm, nor could he see the big picture. He ignored the developing situation in Seattle just has he had paid no attention to the warnings he had received from Peter Navarro. An April 27 article in The Washington Post revealed that those "repeated warnings were conveyed in the President's Daily Briefing...But the alarms failed to register with the President, who routinely skips reading the PDB and at times has shown little patience for even the oral summary he takes two or three times per week."[4]

When President Trump could not be bothered to read or listen to a summary of his February 25 brief, one of his National Security advisors should have told him, "Mr. President, we have a developing situation in Maryland." President Trump should have been forced to acknowledge the part of the Brief which read that at Fort Detrick "the medical intelligence unit raised its warning, that the Coronavirus would become a pandemic within 30 days, from WATCHCON 2—a probable crisis—to WATCHCON 1— an imminent one." This occurred "15 days before the World Health Organization declared the rapidly spreading Coronavirus outbreak to be a global pandemic."[5] I wonder what kind of shape the world would be in today if President Kennedy had ignored repeated warnings about the Missiles of October, if he had told America "it's nothing to worry about," or if he had done nothing and blamed the crisis on President Eisenhower. I wonder too what kind of world Americans will inherit in 2050 based on President Trump's lack of forethought in 2020.

In a classic Far Side cartoon, Gary Larson depicts an intrepid explorer who had sunk into a mass of quicksand, leaving only his wide-brimmed, safari hat floating on the surface. Had he approached the pool from the opposite direction, he would have seen a sign that read "DANGER— QUICKSAND." The cartoon provided an encapsulation of the relationship between President Trump, the President's Daily Briefings, and the Coronavirus. President Trump was blissfully and intentionally ignorant of the threat posed by the Coronavirus. The big difference is that we, not he, are the ones sinking like that unlucky explorer. The President contented himself with watching from a safe distance while we succumbed to a threat he should have spotted and should have assessed as a real and potent danger.

As the death toll climbed in the state of Washington, on March 4, California Governor Gavin Newsome declared a state of emergency in his state because of the two COVID-19 deaths that had occurred in Santa Clara County. Meanwhile in Washington, DC, in a meeting with airline executives, President Trump stated "Some people will have this at a very light level and won't even go to a doctor or hospital, and they'll get better. There are many people like that." This was exactly when hell broke loose in Manhattan.

On March 1, a woman who had returned from Iran was the first positive Coronavirus victim in New York City. On the same day, when the number of New York City cases had risen to eleven, Governor Cuomo declared a state of emergency.

On March 4, more Washington State school districts had closed. Microsoft told its employees that they could stay home even if they were not sick. Amazon employees were told they should work from home. When fifteen people in Washington State had died from COVID-19, Mr. Inslee became the first governor to consider issuing a social distancing mandate. Patty Hayes, the Director for Public Health for Seattle and King County, told reporters "it's a new virus;" "There's no immunity to that;" "There's no vaccine for this:" and "We need to support each other for when we're sick, we stay at home."[6] The next day, Governor Inslee begged Vice President Pence to remove federal restrictions on testing.

By March 6, when the number of New York cases had quadruped, President Trump tweeted about the "new Fake News narrative." Three days later, as the number of positive cases and the death toll grew in New York, California, and Washington, the Dow Jones dropped from twenty-nine thousand to twenty-three thousand, eight hundred and fifty-one. This was Real News for the President, and action was required. Vice President Mike Pence, who on April 28 flaunted the Mayo Clinic's safety policy by brazenly refusing to wear a face covering when he visited that Clinic, infamously announced during a Task Force briefing that a million tests were now available to Americans and that, by the end of the week, that number would increase by another four million. Mr. Pence figured that those numbers would prove that President Trump had the problem well at hand and the stock market would rally upon hearing the good news.

After his visit to the Mayo Clinic, Mr. Pence stated he was unaware of the Clinic's policy. An unnamed Mayo Clinic official confirmed that the Vice President had prior knowledge of the hospital's facemask requirement. Even if he hadn't been so advised, we might have had some vague, last glimmer of hope, misguided as it would prove to be, that the leader of our government's Coronavirus Task Force would not have to be reminded to wear a face covering when making a public appearance—especially in a hospital. It is unlikely that such a decision to enter the facility commando style would have been made by Mr. Pence alone. It is more reasonable to hypothesize that a conversation took place between the Vice President and his Boss, and Mike Pence was told not to wimp out by wearing a mask. Conversely, had he decided on his own to wear a mask, President Trump would have surely taken him to task; Mike would then have hell to pay when a livid President told him he looked stupid wearing a mask because he was not infected.

No one at the Task Force level raised any concerns when those five million tests did not materialize by the end of the week, as Vice President Pence had promised they would. Nearly a month and a half later, questions surfaced about what had happened to those missing tests. At a press conference on April 27, the Vice President told the reporter who had brought this unpleasant fact to light, that the reporter was misinformed. Yes, there were five million tests in a stockpile. He clarified that he did not mean five million tests would be *delivered* or *completed*, he simply meant they would be *available*. Since the mythology of a stockpile worked very well when discussing how many ventilators the Federal Government had on hand, Vice President Pence applied the same conceit to the missing tests. No one would say where the alleged stockpile was located. For all we knew, the ventilators were stacked in a warehouse in Greenville, South Carolina or stashed in a warehouse at the Yucca Mountain Nuclear Waste Repository in Tonopah, Nevada. Wherever those ventilators were hiding, that's where we would find the five million tests, getting riper with each passing day.

Vice President Pence's doubletalk about these mysteriously-missing five million tests was yet another example of the gulf between what President Trump and Vice President Pence publicly espouse, and what they really want to achieve—which is to get re-elected. Knowing he cannot win in November if the economy is in the dumps, President Trump initiated a Three-Part Plan for Re-Election. Part One was comprised of a cheerleading crusade, through which President Trump would preempt primetime Evening News each night with Task Force briefings, where the Good News of the Gospel of Trump would be revealed to a frightened, ill-informed nation. In Part Two of Save the Last Dance for Me, he directed cronies in the Fed to artificially inseminate the stock market with liquidity, thereby inflating the market and improving the Average. Part Three was waiting in the wings—his master plan to re-open the country as quickly as humanly possible. A re-opening would surely cause Wall Street to rebound. If the move was premature, and if the action caused more infections and more deaths, well, that was the cost the American public would pay for doing business. The number of deaths in the United States would soon triple the number of deaths of servicemen during the entire Vietnam conflict, but that fact was A-Ok for the Commander of the New Economy. By following his unconscionably baroque plan to revitalize our economy at the cost of additional lives,

President Trump was confident that on November 4 he would be back in the driver's seat. There would be no reading of the names of the dead, no wall to memorialize the passing of two hundred thousand Americans. We would be left with the knowledge that ninety percent of those lives could have been saved if Mr. Trump had read the President's Daily Briefs.

Chapter Two

Transmission and Incubation

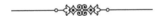

For the past three and a half decades I have worked as a travel agent. I have sold corporate and leisure travel. I went on numerous familiarization trips throughout the world. I travelled to Beijing and Hong Kong, and those China trips gave me an accurate picture of what life is like for the wealthy and the poor in that country. My days of selling leisure travel ended when I purchased and operated my own travel agency for five years. I sold my agency two months prior to 9/11 and from then on, I managed corporate accounts for clients.

For the past twenty-five years, two of those accounts were nonprofit associations funded by the United States Department of Agriculture's Foreign Agriculture Service. Not many travel agents have been as lucky as I have been to retain clients for such a long time; even more fortunately, I have had the luxury of working with clients I like, whose goals I appreciate. These associations were tasked with the mandate to increase the export of United States agriculture products—not commodities, but value-added products like barbeque sauces—to countries throughout the world. The companies that produced these foodstuffs for exporting were small ones, all with fewer than five hundred employees.

My responsibility was to arrange all their travel logistics. I provided airline tickets for association staff members when they conducted missions to other countries. I ticketed groups of foreign buyers when they visited the United States to meet with owners of these small businesses. I generated hotel and ground transportation contracts to accommodate them upon their arrivals. I would often work onsite with these buyers and association staff members once these groups arrived in the United States.

In December 2019, I ticketed approximately twenty of these foreign buyers for an extended stay in the United States. They were due to arrive in Boston on January 31; they would then travel from Boston to New Jersey and then to Pennsylvania, departing from the Philadelphia airport on February 6. Three of these buyers were supposed to originate in Shanghai, Beijing, and Hong Kong.

Brick and mortar travel agents share a responsibility to advise clients when we believe travel is not safe; it is our moral obligation, not part of any contract of carriage. In general, by the end of January the travel agency network was very aware of the Wuhan City Coronavirus problem, and most agents agreed that even though it meant a substantial loss of revenue, advising clients not to travel to or from China by air or cruise ship was the right thing to do.

In my case, this meant telling those three buyers from Beijing, Shanghai, and Hong Kong that they should adjust their travel plans, because we were cancelling their airline and hotel reservations. By disinviting these three buyers, we prevented possible communication of the disease from China to our group. It also allowed us to avoid awkward discussions with the other seventeen buyers, as we attempted to explain why the China buyers were allowed to participate, and why they would be riding in a motorcoach with everyone else for two days of travel between cities. A tangential advantage to cancelling their reservations was accrued, because I could be certain that at least three people on the next United Airlines flights from those cities would not transmit the Coronavirus to three hundred other people on that flight. I figured that one less person on any flight from China meant one less person hosting an easily transmittable disease.

In retrospect, it is remarkable that the travel agent network in the United States recognized that a problem existed and acted upon that recognition weeks before President Trump's order to ban flights from China took effect at 5pm on February 2. Our federal government, with access to more intelligence reports about China than any other country in the world, was woefully late in imposing a ban which was not enforced.

If we turn back the clock to midnight January 1 when China first told the world "we have a problem," and if we examine how many people entered the United States from China from January 1 until mid-April, we come to the shocking recognition that four hundred and thirty thousand airline passengers entered our country from China in that timeframe, including about four thousand entrants arriving directly from Wuhan City. As was made abundantly clear in a comment from World War Z, "the airlines were the perfect delivery system" for spreading a pandemic. To complicate an already-convoluted situation, people who had been exposed to the Coronavirus in China were entering the United States from each of the other countries in the world.

One would have hoped that beginning on February 2, our Customs and Border Protection agency would have been extraordinarily vigilant when questioning each passenger arriving at every international airport in the fifty states. Surely the relative health of individuals permitted to enter from China would be carefully measured and assessed. Given the lethal nature of the virus, CBP officials would certainly take the threat of infection seriously and would implement rigorous screening measures to protect the safety of our borders.

What occurred at our ports of entry was a travesty. Chandler Jurinka, who arrived in Seattle on February 29, told reporters how an immigration officer "hands me my passport and forms and says, 'Oh, by the way, you haven't been to Wuhan, have you...then he says, 'You don't have a fever, right?'" Andrew Wu, who landed at Los Angeles International Airport on March 10, stated ""I was surprised at how lax the whole process was...the guy I spoke to read down a list of questions, and he didn't seem interested in checking out anything." Two weeks later, Sabrina Fitch landed at JFK Airport nonstop from China. She described her "screening" by saying "Besides looking at our passports, they didn't question us like we normally are questioned. So it was kind of weird, because everyone expected the opposite, where you get a lot of questions. But once we filled out the little health form, no one really cared."[1]

These examples and hundreds like them demonstrate once more that it is easy to establish a policy by signing an Executive Order written by an Oval Office lackey. Regarding the next step of policy enforcement, we can assign a low order of probability to the likelihood that our Chief Executive would take commensurate and appropriate steps to enforce such a policy, and that he would hold department heads accountable for any hiccups. Such an expectation is at odds with recent Presidential history. It lies contrary to Mr. Trump's heuristic that talking a big game is better than solving a problem, that a bluff is better than a full house.

Similarly, when President Trump ordered meat processing facilities throughout the nation to re-open on April 29, he did not give the Center for Disease Control and Prevention any authority to enforce the implementation of Coronavirus protection measures in those plants. Consequently, the CDC made suggestions which facility owners could choose to ignore without incurring legal or financial repercussions for their inactions.

Many owners of meat packing plants did just that. If they had followed social distancing measures to protect everyone working in their slaughterhouses, their work force capacity would be cut by seventy-five percent. They would have to open and maintain their entire facility, but they could only expect to kill, process, pack, and ship twenty-five percent of the product. It would be cheaper to remain closed than to open and follow social distancing guidelines.

Since President Trump's Wartime Powers declaration did not mandate that those plants must follow social distancing, the Center for Disease Control's suggestions were watered down beyond recognition. Many owners chose to partially implement protective measures that would allow them to maintain production levels of ninety percent or higher. The health of the workers, the health of the workers' families, the health of all those people who interacted with the workers and their families were at risk. No contact tracing was mandated. President Trump's total interest in the matter began and ended with his signing of the order. No thought was given to visiting a facility, talking to workers, or tracking the rise of positive tests.

His April 29 order virtually condemned to death hundreds of workers in the Smithfield plant in Sioux Falls, in the Tyson facilities in Springdale,

Arkansas and in Waterloo, Iowa, and in a hundred other meat processing plants throughout the country. Like nursing homes, these facilities did not operate in a vacuum. The workers' home communities were infected, the populations of communities with which those people came into contact were infected, and the cycle continued until everyone connected to those meat packing operations through seven degrees of separation were either infected, sick, or dead.

President Trump was afraid that Center for Disease Control officials might present troublesome suggestions to plant owners—and to the American public in general—that would run contrary to his own political agenda. He had grown weary of highfalutin CDC officials making statements that conflicted with his need to present a rosier picture of the times than reality warranted. He took all steps necessary to ensure that the CDC did not have a seat at the table where the biggest game of his career was being played. President Trump had gone all in to muzzle the CDC, expending every chip of political capital in his possession to win a head to head show-down with that organization.

For example, the Center for Disease Control was planning to release a document on May 1, a guide which, according to an AP report, would give "step-by-step advice to local authorities on how and when to re-open." When President Trump's advisors read the guide, the White House reaction was immediate and swingeing. The CDC was told that this helpful and handy guide, produced in the nick of time, "would never see the light of day."[2]

The "shelved report" would have provided the general public with "site-specific decisions related to reopening schools, restaurants, summer camps, churches, day care centers and other institutions" and with "detailed 'decision tree' flow charts" to be used by local officials to help them consider different scenarios. Tips for food service business owners included suggestions to "space tables at least 6 feet (1.8 meters) apart and try to use phone app technology to alert a patron when their table is ready to avoid touching and use of buzzers" and "install sneeze guards at cash registers and avoid having buffets, salad bars and drink stations." Following such guidelines would minimize a national recrudescence of COVID-19, but such a protocol would also have prevented a swift and immediate re-opening of those businesses and social groups. Squelching the guideline was callous move, one which flaunted the President's agenda to re-open at any cost and underlined his seriousness to rid the Executive Branch of the distracting contrariness and needless meddling of so-called "experts."

President Trump should not have viewed the Center for Disease Control as a competitor; the CDC should have been his staunchest ally. Nevertheless, due to his unbridled need to view himself as The Man with the Plan, he forced the CDC to fold its position. A sober awakening was in store for those of us who justifiably but incorrectly imagined the CDC would be our beacon in the dark, an unbiased source of information to guide us in our fight against this pandemic.

This was not the first or only Coronavirus setback we would encounter due to our President's negligence and his ego-driven fantasies, but it certainly was a crucial disappointment. It was another in a long line of cases illustrating our President's misbegotten belief that we should accept everything he tells us at face value. He has implied on many occasions that we should count our blessings and acknowledge on bent knee that we are truly lucky to have him at the helm.

Throughout February, most travel agents, like the public at large, were aware of the extent and compound nature of the problems in China. We continued to sell trips to the rest of the world in February, which was the last month of 2020 in which the unimpeded sale of airline tickets occurred. It was high season, and groups of people bought tickets for Spring Break. Beaches from Miami to Malibu would be filled with partygoers. Many Caribbean and European cruises were sold out. Luxury cruises on ships like the Diamond Princess would captivate three thousand, seven hundred and eleven vacationers on a twenty-seven-day itinerary, stopping at exotic Far East ports from Hong Kong to Yokohama, while being attended to by one thousand and forty-five crew members.

When Italy reported a growing number of Coronavirus-like cases, we advised clients not to travel to Italy. Domestic flights and flights to the rest of the globe were unaffected. There was a scattering of nightly news reports about the Coronavirus, but in the first week of February Americans were told we had nothing to worry about, that cases of Coronavirus infection were few and far between.

When I returned to my home office in Chicago from Philadelphia on February 6, I continued with my routine of planning and ticketing my next group of forty international buyers, who were to attend a global seafood show in Boston, where they would stay for a week in mid-March. Each day the ABC Evening News featured reports on the situation in China and Italy. Concern about the Coronavirus was limited to what was happening in those two countries.

To keep from spreading a disease which we were told was like a flu, Americans were encouraged throughout February to cough into their elbows, and sneeze into a tissue. On February 29, Larry David appeared as Bernie Sanders on Saturday Night Live and shouted that a hand cough was insufficient to defeat a virus—only an elbow cough would ensure the safety of others. He favored the use of a bar of soap and scalding hot water over hand sanitizers, because sanitizers were only ninety-nine-point nine-percent effective. Little did Mr. David know why soap ranked "pretty, pretty good" as a Coronavirus killer. Soap quickly destroys the virus' lipid barrier and within seconds breaks down the structure of the virus.

Thanks to President Trump minimizing of the danger posed by the Coronavirus, the disease was perceived as a joke. Although it was invigorating to find an occasion to laugh, such comments seemed less funny when a person is sick and is perhaps one quick step away from a ventilator.

Political satire, however, is always appreciated. On April 25, the American public was treated to a good example of such satire when Brad Pitt opened Saturday Night Live with a spot-on impersonation of Dr. Fauci explicating President's Trump's attempts to twiddle data as he saw fit. Mr. Pitt's point-counterpoint format decoded the President's paraphrased statements and untangled each of the President's inaccurate conclusions. The monolog illustrated how the President's statements before, during, and after Task Force briefings disserved scientists working around the clock to find solutions to the pandemic.

In the first two weeks of March, though, Larry David's humorous rant was inapposite. The temperament and landscape changed when the numbers of cases of COVID-19 rose in New York, New Jersey, and Illinois.

The immediate problem I faced during the first week of March the imminent arrival of forty buyers I had ticketed to arrive at Boston's Logan Airport from Europe, Asia, Indonesia, South America, and the Caribbean. Airlines were not permitting the refund of any tickets other than those to or from mainland China and Hong Kong. Hotels were not willing to cancel reservations without expecting payment for liquidated damages, because the Coronavirus outbreak was not considered a force majeure. My client accepted the loss of revenue and the concomitant loss of export sales and cancelled the event, thereby securing the safety of those traveling to the United States, of its own staff members coordinating the event, and of the hotel personnel involved in the event.

On that last front, even though the hotels in question did *not* accept the fact that the Coronavirus outbreak was a cause sufficient to warrant a cancellation without a penalty, my client's actions protected the hotel personnel from their own inclinations. By cancelling the event there was no chance of other guests of the hotel or hotel employees being infected by any member of our incoming group. That group would have been in house at midnight on March 13, which was the date that President Trump's ban of European flights became effective. By then there were more than twelve hundred reported cases of COVID-19 in the United States.

Because I work from a home office, my personal contact with other people is limited. I do not commute daily using public transportation, nor do I have many face-to-face meetings with other agents or clients. I meet once a month with a group of authors to hear a guest speaker present a recent publication. The last such meeting I attended was held on March 10.

On March 10 President Trump declared himself immune to COVID-19. Although he had not been tested for COVID-19, he believed the measure was unnecessary. He felt the same way toward the testing the American public in general. He voiced an opinion, unsupported by recent international history or by prevailing facts, when he proclaimed with miracle-worker majesty, "it will go away." It is obvious that President Trump considers himself to be above the law of the land. March 10 was the first time he declared himself immune to the Coronavirus. His failure to wear a mask, his public repudiation of anyone who wore a face covering, and his insistence on outlawing social distancing at his rallies define the presence of a sociopathy—one which was growing in pace with the Coronavirus pandemic.

I live in the Chicago's northwest suburbs, and on that evening of March 10, rather than fight rush hour traffic, I parked my Corolla near a Blue Line train station and took public transportation downtown, to attend my author's meeting. At its conclusion I would return by train to where I had parked my car, and then I would drive to the Countryside Tavern, where I would meet some high school buddies for a few hours of conversation. We like Countryside because the waitresses are cute, and the popcorn is free.

At this point in time, the elbow cough was only instruction given to protect public health. We were weeks away from the beginning of the six-foot guideline for social distancing, and the last time anyone wore a mask in public was October 31. Supplies of hand sanitizers, Clorox wipes, and toilet paper were in abundance wherever one chose to shop. With a quick stop at any drug store or medical supply center, we could purchase as many surgical masks, N-95 masks, latex gloves, hospital gowns, and face shields as we wanted, or as many as could afford.

Each Blue Line train in Chicago is designed to fit about fifty seated passengers. On a busy day, another thirty standing passengers could be crammed into each car. Each plastic bench held two passengers, with two rows of seats facing either forward or backward to the direction of travel, and they were spaced an arm's-length apart, front to back.

Eight seats on each side of the four double doors of each car were designated for seniors and for riders with disabilities. Those seats faced opposite from each other, with about five feet of walkway space separating the two sides.

The car I entered was crowded. Seeing there were no other senior or disabled riders s in the vicinity I selected the priority seat closest to the doors at the rear of the car. Directly across from me sat an attractive thirtysome-thing woman wearing a blue peacoat and a hat.

Without any warning—no coughing, no sniffling, no runny nose—and with her hands resting squarely on her lap, she sneezed. I was not quick enough to react and cover my face, and I clearly felt moisture on my fore-head from her sneeze. There was some grumbling by other passengers, but no one said anything to her until I told her, "Damn, lady, cover your mouth when you do that!" She did not reply—in the finest Chicago tradition, she exhibited no remorse. There was no apology, no "mind your own business," not even a "go fuck yourself" sneer. I wondered how more people upon whom she would sneeze on her way home. I was glad to see her depart the train two stops later at the Logan Square station.

A few weeks later a similar errant sneeze forced a commercial airliner to make an emergency landing, when irate and panicked passengers ganged up on the person in seat Twenty-Two B who may or may not have been a Coronavirus carrier. On March 10 we were not at that stage of readiness. Coughing and sneezing in public raised eyebrows but did not lead to mob actions.

I quickly forgot about The Sneeze; and after my meeting I made an eventless Blue Line commute back to Harlem Avenue. I walked to my car and drove to Countryside. It was an enjoyable gathering, and when we left Countryside, we had no idea that this would be our last meeting for quite some time.

Responding to the alarming report that there were ninety-three confirmed cases of COVID-19 in Illinois, Governor J.B. Pritzker ordered all ten Illinois casinos to close, effective March 13. He followed up that action on March 15, when he said that all bars and restaurants in the state would be closed at end of the next day. Pritzker pulled no punches when he stated, "The time for persuasion and public appeals is over. The time for action is here. This is not a joke. No one is immune to this, and you have an obligation to act in the best interests of all the people of this state."[3] Such a bold statement did not endear our Democratic governor to the President, whose day-in, day-out goal was to minimize, not emphasize, the seriousness of the threat. Nor did Governor Pritzker win himself many friends in the White House when he tweeted, "the federal government needs to get its s@#t together!"

Closed casinos meant a massive loss of revenue for the state, and for the villages, townships, and counties that depended on gaming revenue to pay for essential services; I took Pritzker's words and actions to heart. I told my clients who were on flights to or from Chicago that we needed to cancel those air reservations and issue refunds when possible. Aware of the constant flow of traffic at O'hare Airport on a normal day, none of my clients wanted to experience what could very well be a frenzied crowd in TSA lines, nor were they anxious to endure the hours of waiting while flights to LaGuardia, Newark, and Seattle were delayed.

Refunds were not easy to come by because, like the Boston hotel, airlines did not consider the Coronavirus outbreak to be an adequate reason to warrant issuing refunds. By the time our federal ban of flights to and from European cities came into play, airlines had become so strapped for cash that, for the first time to my knowledge, they unilaterally declined to issue refunds for refundable electronic tickets.

Instead of refunds, airlines would allow re-scheduling of flights without a penalty if that re-scheduling occurred before the end of 2020. Airline executives rightly and callously predicted that many, perhaps a majority of those passengers might not need to travel to the destination they had selected for March 2020 travel in 2021, allowing each airline to capture one hundred percent of the revenue from the original transaction. To the advantage of the airline, any new ticket that was issued in exchange for a previous eticket would be subject to higher fares applicable at the time of the new transaction. It was also likely that many passengers would forget about travelling, and the monies paid for those etickets constituted an additional revenue stream. Airline forecasters knew that a fair to middling number of original passengers would be so disgusted by the new "no refund" policy that they would swear never to travel on that airline again, which would generate an additional revenue flow.

A quick check of Facebook postings and tweets from disgruntled passengers during the months of March-April 2020 shows that this fourth line of reasoning was a completely accurate airline prediction. Passengers were not complacent about the airlines' highhanded treatment of loyal customers. Passengers also wondered if our government would add insult to injury by forcing taxpayers to foot the bill to bail out the airline industry once the pandemic had ended. The bank bailout of 2008 attested to the validity of that supposition.

There is a further reason why we should not pity the airlines for its loss of sales revenue and for the drastic drop in the price of AA, UA, and DL stocks. The decline of jet fuel prices—lower than they were in the 1960s—has allowed airlines to buy fuel futures at rock-bottom prices. We can be certain that those savings will *not* be passed on to customers in 2021. Higher fuel prices in 2021 will allow airlines to add fuel surcharges to the cost of an eticket, with passengers paying more for fuel previously purchased at discounted prices. This is exactly how the airlines have operated for the past half-century, and we have no reason to believe the Coronavirus pandemic will cause the chief executive officers of those three airlines to have a change of heart.

When I returned home late on March 10, I set aside thoughts of the Sneeze. There was no reason to dwell on what had happened that night on the Blue Line near Jefferson Park. I had committed to giving a lecture and doing a book signing event at a local library on March 12, and I needed to prepare my presentation. Before I went to the library on the Twelfth, I stopped at a drug store and bought a package of menthol cough drops. I was about to speak and respond to questions for about two hours, and I had noticed that I had been coughing frequently earlier that day. I thought that since it had been rainy, I was coughing due to change in weather. The cough drops proved to be an effective remedy, and the event was successful. I made some new friends, which was the best part of the endeavor.

When I awoke the next morning, my head felt fuzzy. I concluded that this disorientation was a sign of a cold coming on, which I half-expected to happen because I had been coughing more frequently than normal. I didn't expect that that these symptoms were related in any way to the Coronavirus, especially since most of the cases in the United States were located in New York and I hadn't had any contact lately with anyone from that state. Had these symptoms manifested themselves two weeks or a month later, my reaction would have been different. I would have experienced a higher level of apprehension, and I would have been concerned that as late as March 29, no public testing for COVID-19 was offered in Illinois.

By March 17, my revenue from the sale of airline tickets had been declined significantly. I was not concerned, because Governor Pritzker's order to close business was limited to two weeks, and I had survived a much longer period of sales inactivity after 9/11. I figured that the Coronavirus was like SARS and MERS and the Avian Flu, all of which temporarily short-circuited my sales. I expected that the Coronavirus would have a similar, temporarily negative effect on my ability to conduct business.

Truth be told, by the third week of March I did not feel much like working, and I was grateful for the lull in business. Most vendors with whom I dealt were experiencing a similar lull. In what seemed to be a random fashion, companies in Illinois told employees to stay at home if they felt sick. Soon that suggestion would be amended to a common directive to "stay at home even if you aren't sick." By March 19 I realized I belonged in the first of those two categories. I started taking my temperature on March 22 and found to my chagrin that I was cooking at one hundred and two degrees.

It was at this point that I first considered the real possibility that I was suffering from COVID-19. I began to do research online to find out what were the symptoms and the typical progression of the disease. I learned that the most common symptoms were coughing, stuffiness, fever, and sneezing. On those counts I was batting four for four.

I became at best distracted, at worst obsessed with trying to figure out how this could have happened to me. I had heard somewhere that only point-three percent of the population would be affected, and I wondered how I could have been so unlucky. I did not know if that estimate was entirely accurate, but I was aware that the odds of contracting the Coronavirus were remote.

I naturally wondered if I was being punished for past misdeeds. I never claimed to have lived a saintly life. When I was in my thirties, after my first book was published, I rode a wave of misconstrued invincibility. My lifestyle had been profligate. I drank to excess on occasion. I treated some women selfishly. I gambled recklessly and had played the stock market as though I were an insider. Maybe I had not been a good enough teacher or coach. Perhaps I had unknowingly caused harm to others. I wondered if these and countless other transgressions come home to roost.

I knew that such speculation did not help matters. I was aware that in all probability the cause of my illness was not mystical; it was the result of my coming into close and unintended physical contact with a carrier of the Coronavirus. I also recognized that because there were so many possible opportunities for transmission, trying to figure out how I had been infected was a losing proposition. At the same time, I held on to the hope that what I was experiencing was not an incipient stage of COVID-19. I conceded that hoping not to have COVID-19 was ineffective and constituted a form of denial.

I wanted to believe I had not been infected with the Coronavirus because I had heard that if I had contracted COVID-19, the odds of me dying from it were pretty low, *unless* I was an older person who had any underlying medical problems. My concern was that I was of age and I had a slew of underlying medical conditions. Twelve years earlier I was diagnosed with mild cardiac disease. I had two angiograms, and although stents were contraindicated, I was put on eighty milligrams of atorvastatin and one low-dose aspirin, per night. I take Lisinopril to combat hypertension, Omeprazole for acid reflux, and when I dine at restaurants I have an Epipen on hand because I am allergic to garlic, and I need to be prepared if there is cross-contamination in what I had been assured was a garlic-free entrée. I try to eat healthily; I cannot remember the last time I had a McDonald's or Burger King hamburger and french fries. I have a family history of heart disease and cancer.

I lived in a suburb of Seattle for five years, and during that time I began to experience pain in my extremities. I did not pay much attention to the pain until I began to stumble because I couldn't lift the front of my left foot, and I had difficulty holding down chords with my left hand when I played guitar. I underwent a lengthy series of electromyography tests—shocks, really—administered and measured by neurologists at the Virginia Mason Hospital in Seattle. After a spinal tap was performed, I was diagnosed as having CIDP, which stood for chronic inflammatory demyelinating polyneuropathy. What this meant in everyday English was that my immune system was attacking the myelin, which is the insulating cover of the nerves. If the symptoms progressed to acute, the condition would be designated as Guillain-Barre syndrome.

Two radically different forms of treatment were offered to mitigate the chronic symptoms: megadoses of the corticosteroid Prednisone to suppress my immune system were possible, or weekly infusions of immunoglobulin could be used to boost my immune system's response to CIDP.

The Prednisone path had the huge disadvantages of causing weight gain, glaucoma, fluid retention, elevated blood pressure, cardiac impairment, mood swings, memory dysfunctions, confusion, and delirium. These were not possible side effects like the ones shown in fine print at the end of a television commercial for a new Big Pharm designer drug. These were the inevitable consequences of taking so much Prednisone. The advantage was that the drug quickly and effectively masked any CIDP pain I would experience, and it should halt the demyelinating process.

Immunoglobulin infusions were not stroll in the park. It would take between four and five hours to complete each set of infusions, depending on the rate of the drip. Five daily treatments were required once a month, to continue until the CIDP symptoms decreased and hopefully ended for good. The first week of treatments would require a hospital stay, which would facilitate a quick move to the ICU if a severe enough reaction to the infusion presented itself. After that, if all went well, the infusions could be done on an outpatient basis. The disadvantage was that my heart's reaction to the treatment could not be predicted. The advantage was that, if it worked, the infusions would repair damage done by CIDP and the symptoms would dissipate.

My neurologist recommended the infusions. I would be part of the thirty-nine percent of CIDP patients treated in this manner. I agreed. On the positive side, this meant I would not need another spinal tap. Anyone who has undergone that proceed can understand why one spinal tap in a lifetime is one too many.

During the first week of the infusions my reactions were severe. I was given Zofran to lessen nausea, but my stomach was constantly jumpy, and I had no appetite. I experienced chills and had an elevated temperature. Looking back, I realize how mild those symptoms were, compared to how severely out of whack COVID-19 would throw my system. After five months of this infusion regimen, follow-up EMG tests indicated that the demyelination had ceased, and the treatments could end. I had recovered full use of my arms and legs; to date the condition has not recurred.

I tried not to dwell on my medical history. There was nothing I could do to change the past. I had more immediate concerns. One source of worry was my cat. I did not wish to transmit COVID-19, if I had the disease, to Sonia. She had inherited the respiratory problem known as Feline Infectious Peritonitis, for which there was no cure. The disease caused breathing difficulties. I felt less troubled about the possibility of infecting her when I heard Dr. Fauci state that such a transmission was unlikely. I had read online that FIP was caused by a form of coronavirus, which led me to conclude, quite unscientifically, that if she already had the virus, she could not get it again. Over the weeks since March 10 I noticed her condition had not changed, which was an encouraging sign. Looking at the situation from another angle, I thought, again without any shred of evidence, that her not getting sick meant maybe I did not have COVID-19.

I had no luck finding any information, anecdotal or clinical, about the daily progression of COVID-19 symptoms. This was a discouraging and shocking fact. I wondered why there were not stories about what tens of thousands of Americans were experiencing. Hadn't people adequately recovered from the disease to tell their tales? I asked myself why no doctors had clarified what to expect and what to do about it if we had COVID-19. I had been watching MSNBC regularly and I had not seen any such story. I needed to know how long my fever would last. I had a hundred other questions to which I could find no answer. I wondered if or when the fever breaks, does that mean the disease has ended. I did not know if a dry cough was a good or bad indicator. I had no index to tell if I was getting COVID-19 pneumonia. I wanted to know why my symptoms were so unlike those that came with any flu I experienced in the past.

I could not get a flu shot due to a possible CIDP immune interaction. Each time I did have a flu, the cycle consisted of chills, headache, a fever, sneezing and stuffiness, dry coughing, a sweaty night when the fever broke, followed by lessening congestion and wet coughing, There was no shortness of breath that I could recall, and my headaches persisted for a day at most.

By the fourth week of March 2020, though, I had an elevated temperature that would last for several days, then it would abate, only to return a day or two later. Since taking aspirin is the recommended form of treatment for a fever, I took a low dose aspirin every five hours, which resulted in lowering my temperature by two degrees. I consumed bag after bag of cough suppressants, but the relief was temporary. My headaches and my shortness of breath were constant.

I had heard stories on television about what ventilator-assisted breathing meant, and it was a scary proposition. Patients are intubated and another tube is inserted into the bladder. Once the venting starts, teams of medical assistants monitor the progression on a 24/7 basis. A schedule of rotations of body positions is followed to help with breathing. Eventually the tubes are removed and breathing with the help of an external oxygen supply continues for as long as necessary. After a while, oxygen is no longer required because the patient's lungs have begun to heal, and the patient is released to go home. That was Plan A, and it was the best-case scenario. Unfortunately, it was not what usually happens to patients.

Plan B involved a more common and terrifying scenario. Once you go into the hospital and are put on a ventilator, you do not come out. If there is a dignified way to die, this is not it. You are out of contact with loved ones, friends, and relatives. Up until the time you mercifully slip into a coma and die, you are aware that what is happening to you is not good. The only conscious action you can take is to pray to God you will be spared from this condition. Those prayers are always answered, even if the answer is not what most patients would like to hear.

Putting aside such sobering thoughts, on the morning of March 26 I called a local hospital. I explained my symptoms and said, "I think I should be tested for COVID-19." The reply I heard was surprising, but it should not have been unexpected. I knew that New York had problems with testing, and televised reports indicated that tests in the New York metropolitan areas were in short supply. But as is often the case with COVID-19, you do not understand that what is happening to many other people in faraway cities is happening to you. Denial is a formidable defense mechanism.

I was told by an emergency room attendant that I could be tested. First, I needed a referral from my doctor. No problem, I figured; my GP was always ready to help with whatever symptoms and ailments I reported to him. I knew that when I left a message, I would receive a call back in less than an hour. A referral would be faxed immediately to the correct number. The emergency room person to whom I was speaking added a second wrinkle; she said I would also need an authorization from IDPH, the Illinois Department of Public Health. I thanked the woman and ended the call.

For the rest of that Thursday, on the hour every hour I tried to contact the IDPH by phone. Because the website was down much of that time, calling was the only option. On the few occasions when the line was not busy, I heard an automated voice telling me that if this was an emergency I should hang up and dial 911.

Upon hearing that disclaimer I wondered who in their right mind would not call 911 if a life-threatening and immediate medical problem had arisen. If I were stabbed in a back alley at 73rd and Hermitage where I grew up, for example, I would not call the Illinois Department of Public Health for assistance as I bled out. Then I heard a disembodied voice state that "due to the large number of calls, all representatives are busy." That was okay with me. I would wait until hell froze over with my phone on speaker if it resulted in me getting the referral that the hospital required.

The other shoe dropped when I heard the voice which I had grown to dislike intensely tell me that if I was calling about COVID-19 I should visit the website for answers to common questions. After pressing zero four times, I was told "due to the high volume of calls, please call back at another time."

I have always used my frustration with computerized call centers and large volumes of calls to motivate me to be more persistent, and so for the rest of that Thursday I channeled my anger and repeatedly called that same number, crazily hoping that one of those times I would get lucky. I was employing the same logic that leads people to purchase Powerball lottery tickets twice a week. I knew that my chances of obtaining the required authorization were about the same as winning that Powerball or Mega-Million Grand Prize, but I was willing and desperate enough to plop down my two dollars and cross my fingers. I did not win the brass ring that day, or any day in March when I attempted to call the Illinois Department of Public Health.

Panic about my situation began to creep in when I drew the only reasonable conclusion I could, which was that I was just as stymied as everyone else in America who needed to be tested for COVID-19 at a time when no such test was available. Panic made me irritable. I began to resent people who complained that social distancing kept them at home. I hated hearing President Trump say that our southern border was protected from the

Coronavirus by two or five hundred miles of solid wall. It reminded me of ancient thinking when, during the Thracian Wars, Greek warriors arranged themselves in a shield wall to protect the King. President Trump's wall certainly was not metaphorical, it was not the shield that love provides, the one that Deep Purple had in mind when they sang that we should "trust in The Shield." I was afraid I would jump out my skin if I heard President Trump claim once more that "I built the greatest economy in the history of the world."

Although I am not a stupid person, I could not understand how our President could state that the Coronavirus would simply disappear. The sheer incomprehensibility of his words further angered me. I felt beleaguered, worn down by his claims that he alone was responsible for everything good that had happened in this country since President Obama's term in office. I wondered what those good things were, and what actions of his constituted achieving all of them. I questioned why the Coronavirus was being politicized by him at a time when, with each passing hour, the number of cases of COVID-19 increased and the body count in the United States mounted.

We were living in a time of crisis, and we needed a leader like Franklin Roosevelt, John F. Kennedy, or Barack Obama. We needed a person who understood the suffering of the average American and who acted with clear intelligence and with an abundance of caution. We required someone in Office who would act decisively to protect the life and freedom of every citizen. Instead we had Mr. I Take No Responsibility, a President who believes that when Harry Truman said "Inside this room, the buck stops" he was referring to a dollar bill.

I was embittered by the fact that so many young people, whose experience with a virus was limited to what happened to their computers after they visited too many dodgy websites, thought that with the right Norton software this virus could be eradicated. I was tired of hearing billionaires like Liz and Dick Uihlein, owners of the shipping company Uline, calling for an immediate resumption of business as usual. It did not matter to these wealthy Trump supporters how many people would die making sure a dozen Uline containers left the Port of Long Beach as scheduled and arrived in Hong Long on time.

I was worried that if I had been infected with the Coronavirus, the people I had been in contact with on March 10 and March 12 might soon be getting sick, if they were not ill already. Ultimately I was afraid that because there was no cure for the virus and no vaccine available in the foreseeable future, I would soon be dead, and the dreams I had of retiring to an island in the Caribbean where I could live peacefully and write books about the history of classic rock would never be actualized. I tried not dwell on that primal possibility—I worked hard to maintain the optimism and joy in life that had so far defined my existence. I would apply the same Cartesian logic that I had always used to solve problems to resolve the Coronavirus threat I faced. I would reduce the larger issue of recovery down to its discrete parts, and in doing so, I would surely find a way to navigate these unsettling waters. And I would pray that God would help me find a way out of this predicament. Those were the tools I had on hand to fight the disease. I felt a deep-seated certainty that these tools would be formidable enough to cope with COVID-19.

I admit I was in a bit of a quandary regarding how I would get tested. Testing options seemed limited. They existed in a sphere with which I was unfamiliar. The best plan I could envision was to get in my car and drive to Springfield and not leave the Capitol Building until I convinced some clerk at the Department of Health to authorize a test. Coronavirus testing without IDPH authorization had begun for city and state officials and health care providers, but things still looked bleak for the average joe needing a test.

The horizon changed when on Saturday, March 28, WGN Television News announced that, with the help of the United States Army, Chicago had begun operating a drive-through testing site at 6959 Forest Preserve Drive. It was location that had previously housed a vehicle emissions testing center.

COVID-19 tests would be administered on first come, first serve basis. The problem this posed for me is that when it opened on March 29, testing would be limited to health care providers and first responders. Illinois officials amended the requirements later on that Sunday and stated that starting on March 30, anyone over age sixty-five who had Coronavirus symptoms would be permitted to join the line to receive one of the two hundred and fifty tests that could be given each day, according to federal restrictions. The facility would open at 9 a.m.

Testing was by no means signified a cure, but it was a step in the right direction. It meant that anyone who tested positive would be self-quarantined and contact tracing could begin.

Knowing what happens in Chicago on the first day that anything opens in our city, I thought that before I joined the crowd, I would watch what happened on March 30. Televised reports at 9 a.m. on the 30th included helicopter footage depicting a line of automobiles that extended for two miles. The queue of cars snaked down Forest Preserve Drive west to Harlem Avenue, south to Irving Park Road, and then east on Irving Park. The line did not seem to move in the thirty seconds of footage that I saw. It was the longest static parade of cars I had witnessed since May 21, 2019 when I waited for hours to leave the parking lot of the Hollywood Casino Amphitheater after seeing The Who's "Movin' On" concert.

The <u>WGN</u> reporter provided the crucial bit of information I was hoping he would include. He mentioned that cars had arrived to get in line as early as 4 a.m. Based on that observation, I formulated a plan which had a high probability of succeeding. No matter how poorly I felt, I was going to win the lottery and get that test the day, allowing me to confront a reality I would rather have avoided. I understood that knowing is better than not knowing. Wishing and pretending that I did not have COVID-19 was a loser's game. Although an enemy might be "unseen," with available technology it could be detected.

Chapter Three

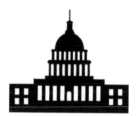

The Blame Game

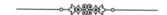

A scapegoat is a handy commodity when plans go terribly awry. Its relative importance increases as the unwillingness or inability to perceive reality correctly increases. Such was the equation that described President's Trump's public persona at the beginning of April 2020. His clay pigeons were China, the World Health Organization, President Obama, Democratic members of House of Representatives and the Senate, and governors of states and territories.

President Trump had delivered a consistent message that the federal approach to the Coronavirus pandemic was a complete success, that every outcome had been anticipated and met with aplomb. When bumps in the road were encountered, one or several of the above groups of miscreants and everyone else in the world, except for residents of the White House, were the guilty parties.

On April 2, <u>CCN</u>.com reported that "Donald Trump and his supporters have been focused on shifting the blame to China for the coronavirus crisis in the U.S."[1] On April 7, President Trump broadened his complaints about

China by incriminating the World Health Organization. He tweeted, "The W.H.O. really blew it. For some reason, funded largely by the United States, yet very China centric. We will be giving that a good look. Fortunately I rejected their advice on keeping our borders open to China early on. Why did they give us such a faulty recommendation?"

While beating a dead horse with his self-laudatory and untrue "I closed the borders very early" claim, the President continued to confound native English speakers by inventing the term "China-centric." The term did not represent as egregious misuse of the lexicon as "covfefe," "Nambia," "perhsps," and "monummt," or in his preference for designer slurs like "bad hombres." In a perfect world this new "China-centric" adjective will not find its way into the Oxford English Dictionary.

On April 14, the Center for American Progress stated that "Trump attempts to shift blame on China by regularly highlighting the ban he placed on travel from China—despite the ineffectiveness of that ban." Its article concluded that "Instead of using every lever at his disposal to help Americans, President Trump, along with his supporters, is whipping up an anti-China frenzy to obscure what may be the biggest leadership failure this nation has ever seen."[2] The article included a quote from political messaging specialist Professor Lisa Burns, who stated, "The default was to go back to the China excuse and deflecting to China...When you're playing to a base, looking for that red meat, scapegoating is one of your best strategies."

Forgetting for a moment that four years prior, President Trump had solicited China's assistance in securing him a favorable outcome in the 2016 election, on April 14 the Trump campaign sent out a fundraising email stating that "China has been lying and doing everything they can to cover up the spread of Covid-19 in their country. It's absolutely disgraceful and we can't stand by and do nothing."[3] The RNC did not mention the fact that when the Donald Trump went hand in hat seeking China's support in the upcoming 2016 election, he encouraged President Xi to establish concentration camps to "re-educate" the Muslim Uighur population of Xinjiang, using forced labor and cattle prods as pedagogical tools.

On that same date, Intelligencer magazine asserted, "Trump is trying to get voters to stop thinking of the coronavirus as a public-health problem, and instead imagine it as a foreign-policy confrontation, with the important quality of leadership being a willingness to offend China."[4] Because President Trump believes that blame for the pandemic is intimately connected to the likelihood of him defeating Former Vice President Joe Biden in November, President Trump politicized the Coronavirus pandemic by releasing an ad claiming that "Biden protected China's feelings while China cripples America."[5] In Tulsa, President Trump took the Biden blame a step further, stating that "Sleepy Joe" Biden was controlled by "leftwing radicals," by a "leftwing mob," and by "radical maniacs."

President Trump's staunch media ally, Fox News, featured a story describing how Senator Chris Murphy had told CNN's Anderson Cooper "The reason that we're in the crisis that we are today is not because of anything that China did, is not because of anything the WHO did. It's because of what this president did...It's because he didn't take this virus seriously. We weren't going to be able to keep every case out of the United States, but we didn't have to have tens of thousands of people dying."[6] Criticism of the President did not occur frequently on Fox News: amazingly, the story recounted the Senator's belief that President Trump was guilty "of shifting blame for the extent of the Coronavirus pandemic onto China and the World Health Organization instead of accepting responsibility." The next day President Trump ended the United States' funding of the World Health Organization.

In his never-ending search for an additional way to distract attention from his failure to manage America's Coronavirus outbreak, President Trump held Congress's feet to the fire. Because of its failure to act quickly and decisively to approve his new political appointments, on April 15 President Trump stated he would invoke Article 2, Section 2, Clause 3 of the Constitution. Congress would be adjourned to allow him to make recess appointments. He announced "We have a tremendous number of people that have to come into government and now more so than ever before because of the virus...If the House will not agree to that adjournment, I will exercise my constitutional authority to adjourn both chambers of Congress."

The significance and extraordinary implications of such a move cannot be underestimated. Historian Michael Beschloss reminded Americans that "No President in history has ever used the Constitutional power to adjourn Congress...Wilson, Taft and FDR were all urged to adjourn Congress and all refused."[7] When Mitch McConnel refused to get on board with President Trump's astounding threat, the President tweeted "They know they've been warned and they've been warned right now. If they don't approve it, then we're going to go this route and we'll probably be challenged in court and we'll see who wins." To avoid such a conflict in the middle of a pandemic, both the House and the Senate extended their recesses until May 4.

On April 16 the President said "I'm getting tired of China." Meanwhile, the Republican National Committee blamed House Speaker Nany Pelosi for inadequate Paycheck Protection Plan funding. The RNC stated "The Paycheck Protection Program ran out of money this morning because Democrats, led by Nancy Pelosi, blocked the necessary $250 billion replenishment for the program that Congressional Republicans tried to deliver." Trump campaign responder Steve Guest called Ms. Pelosi "Nancy Antoinette" because she had given viewers a tour of her kitchen when she appeared on The Late, Late Show. Guest's name calling piggybacked on a long line of audacious Trump statements about Pelosi. On April 15 President Trump boasted, "They didn't want our borders closed. They're criticizing me for closing the border. I did that very early. By the way, I did that very early while Nancy Pelosi was trying to have in San Francisco parties in Chinatown because she thought it would be great."

On the morning of the Seventeenth of April, President Trump tweeted that the number of deaths in China were "far higher than the U.S., not even close!" He took a vacation from his China-centric world to voice his support for everyone who protested social distancing. He also had a bone to pick with New York Governor Andrew Cuomo.

Regarding the protestors, President Trump he tweeted it was time to "LIBERATE MICHIGAN," "LIBERATE MINNESOTA," and to "LIBERATE VIRGINIA, and save your great 2nd Amendment. It is under siege!" A tweet directed at Governor Cuomo stated "We have given New York far more money, help and equipment than any other state, by far, & these great men & women who did the job never hear you say thanks...Your numbers are not good. Less talk and more action!" Clearly Andrew Cuomo was chastised out of jealousy, since Cuomo's daily press conferences were popular because they were fact-based, well-reasoned, immediately understandable, and were delivered in a sympathetic tone and down-to-earth manner. By comparison, the appeal of each of President Trump's Coronavirus Task Force briefings had dwindled, languishing in a sorry mix of sententious rhetoric and press corps traduction, hosted by a president who was all talk and no action.

On April 18, a nonplussed President revealed that "Our relationship with China was good until they did this." On April 19 <u>Business Insider</u> reported that "President Donald Trump has claimed that China may have allowed the Coronavirus to spread deliberately" and that "top advisers claim attacking Beijing may be the best way for the President to save his job."[8] During that evening's press conference, President Trump stated, "It could have been stopped in China before it started and it wasn't, and the whole world is suffering because of it." Later he would imply in tweets that the Coronavirus was a new Chinese bioweapon.

On April 20, before President Trump announced his ban on immigration to the United States, he returned to attacking Governor Cuomo in tweets, writing that "Cuomo ridiculously wanted 40 thousand Ventilators. We gave him a small fraction of that number, and it was plenty." Next, he compared the 1917 flu pandemic to the Coronavirus outbreak, momentarily forgetting that the year of the Spanish Flu outbreak was 1918, which was the year that the Spanish flu claimed the life of his grandfather Frederick.

President Trump should have avoided blaming China for anything on April 21 when members of the U.S.-China Economic and Security Review Commission reported that his continued China-bashing "raises the possibility that implementation could be disrupted."[9] This "implementation" referred to President Trump's two-years-in-the-making-but never-out-of-the-gate, multi-billion-dollar trade deal with China. This oft-touted bonanza was to be symbolic of the re-opening of our economy. Unfortunately, his errant tweets, the White House remarks, and his blaming China for what happened in the USA under his tutelage were counterproductive to his goal of artfully closing the China deal.

This paradigm was another illustration of the President's inability to learn from past mistakes. In this case, the lesson that was *not* heeded was a simple one—that his words have long-term, regrettable consequences. He was acutely aware that at the April 21 Task Force briefing he should not mention the word China or any similar referent like "tariff" or "made in." If he did so, surely some wiseacre reporter would ask him, "President Trump, about your China trade deal—how's that working out for you?" The rest of the Corps would chime in and soon our dyspeptic President would have dug himself into a deeper hole than he had previously imagined possible.

Instead of keeping his mouth shut about China and mentioning every other country in the world *except* China, he could not restrain himself from mentioning you know what. When speaking about closing borders to immigrants, he could have gotten away with mentioning a country like Mexico or Italy or Croatia, and he would have stood on relatively firm ground. Instead, like a dog with a bone, he blurted out "like China or some of the other ones that I've shut down."

His comment could not have been well-received in Beijing. President Trump may have believed that it was a smart public relations move to repeat that banishing China from the United States would help him win the war with "the Invisible Enemy," but he threw caution to the wind, perhaps not realizing that losing a trade deal such as this one would not further his goal of revitalizing the economy. In a sense, he was like General Jack D. Ripper in <u>Dr. Strangelove</u>, a man who could not keep from assisting in his own demise.

Throughout the course of these daily briefings, reporters had learned the hard way that it is best not to challenge the President's statements on semantic grounds. It would be fruitless for them to point out on this occasion that, like all viruses, the Invisible Enemy is easily observed by using an electron microscope. The Coronavirus did not possess a Claude Rains secret invisibility formula, nor was it an abstract concept like Communism. His use of this idiomatic expression was reckless because it shrouded the pandemic in mysterious and foreboding airs at exactly the time when Americans struggled to understand the clear and present dangers of COVID-19.

President Trump had bigger fish than China to fry on April 22. In a series of terrible ironies, first he planted a tree to celebrate Earth Day, while his Koch Brother cronies amassed greater fortunes by cutting down trees to produce the "wood chips" necessary to operate their biomass facilities under the auspices of Green Energy. Next, while those American forests were being plundered, the President announced he would re-open our National Parks. Visitors would have ringside seats to watch Komatsu D575A and Caterpillar D11 bulldozers ravage the previously virgin forests in and near White Mountain, Joshua Tree, and Yellowstone National Parks, for example, while they sat at campfires and infected each other with COVID-19. Finally, the President said it was "beautiful" and "encouraging" to watch individual states re-open—unless one of those states was Georgia. Governor Brian Kemp was about to open barber shops for business, forgetting that he had to be careful when addressing the topic of coiffure when Mr. Trump was in earshot.

As if a question about hair styling was not enough to piss off an already agitated Commander in Chief, on this same evening President Trump learned that Iran had launched a satellite into orbit, one which was conceivably a part of an Iranian space weapons program. Upon hearing the unsupported allegation of Iranian space weaponry circling the Earth, President Trump went ballistic in his attempt to resolve a different Iranian incursion, one to which he could respond in force. He could not shoot down a nonexistent satellite, but he sure as hell was not going to countenance Iranian gunboats near the Harry S. Truman Carrier Strike Group

President Trump tweeted, "I have instructed the United States Navy to shoot down and destroy any and all Iranian gunboats if they harass our ships at sea." Next he told reporters "We don't want their gunboats surrounding our boats and traveling around our boats and having a good time. We're not going to stand for it...They'll shoot them out of the water." The New York Times wrote that President Trump made these comments "without citing any specific incident."[10] The last Iran gunboat incident had occurred a week prior, when our ships "used a variety of nonlethal means to warn off the Iranian boats, and they eventually left."[11] Since the President has a demonstrated inability to juggle two concepts at the same time without getting confused, he was most likely thinking "shoot down and destroy satellite" since gunboats can be sunk but cannot be shot down.

Two other states that were primed and ready to re-open were Florida and Texas. On April 17 Florida's Governor Ron DeSantis declared that it was time to resume beach volleyball; the next day crowds swarmed the Gulf and Atlantic side beaches. It was an event about which Forbes commented,

"Meanwhile, on Twitter, **#FloridaMorons** is the no. 1 trending hashtag in the U.S."[12] Two weeks later, although the number of positive Coronavirus tests had spiked, the beaches remained open. Two months later, the beaches were closed, because the number of positive Coronavirus tests had continued to rise.[13]

Texas Governor Greg Abbott and Lt. Governor and Lt. Governor Dan Patrick proved themselves to be true balance-sheet believers. They wanted to re-open a state which they thought should never have been closed. Lt. Governor Patrick made national news when he told Tucker Carlson, "At the end of January, Dr. Fauci, who I have great respect for, said this wasn't a big issue. Three weeks later, we were gonna lose two million people. Another few weeks later, it was one to two-hundred thousand. Now it's under 60,000, and we've had the wrong numbers, the wrong science. And I don't blame them, but let's face [the] reality of where we are. In Texas, we have 29 million people, [and] we've lost 495. Every life is valuable, but 500 people out of 29 million and we're locked down. And we're crushing the average worker, we're crushing small business, we're crushing the markets, we're crushing this country. And what I said when I was with you that night, *there are more important things than living*, and that's saving this country for my children, and my grandchildren, and saving this country for all of us. And I don't wanna die. Nobody wants to die. But we gotta take some risks, and get back in the game, and get this country back up and running."[14]

The consequences of prematurely and recklessly re-opening Texas were dire. On March 4 the Texas state health department reported its first positive case of COVID-19. By Monday, May 4, "approximately thirty-three thousand Texans had tested positive for the coronavirus."[15] Texas had a full complement of prisons, nursing homes, and meat processing facilities. Inmates at its prisons and patients at its nursing home were not venturing out into the community, but staff members at both facilities certainly were. Employees at its meat-packing plants had free rein to go swimming at a Padre Island beach, to shop at one of Texas' nearly sixteen thousand retail stores, or to join hands with other spectators at the Orca Encounter at SeaWorld in San Antonio. Even if the employees were asymptomatic when they left their workplaces, there was no guarantee they were not carriers.

What we *can* guarantee is that if the state had remained closed, if social distancing measures were strictly enforced, and if Texas did not have one of the lowest numbers of tests performed, there would have been less than thirty two thousand, three hundred and thirty-one new cases of COVID-19 in that same timeframe. By mid-July, after several rounds of opening and closing, Texas had two hundred and sixty-five thousand cases of COVID-19, resulting in over three thousand deaths. Five hundred deaths were acceptable losses for Lt. Governor Patrick. Three thousand bereaved Texas families did not consider the deaths of their loved ones to be acceptable.

News cycles define President Trump's words and actions. He suspected that someday, assertions of China's culpability would get old. He had run the full gamut with China. For example, on January 24 he had tweeted "China has been working very hard to contain the Coronavirus. The United States greatly appreciates their efforts and transparency. It will all work out well. In particular, on behalf of the American People, I want to thank President Xi!" His remarks on May 29 illustrate the incongruity of his position vis-a-vis China; he stated, "The world is now suffering as a result of the malfeasance of the Chinese government." Having played both ends against the middle, it was time for him to call out other parties as causes and contributors to the uncontrolled spread of the Coronavirus in the United States.

Governors of the United States—the ones viewed as enemies by the Trump Administration—were next in line to have bull's eyes painted on their backs. These were the Democratic governors, the ones to whom President Trump referred when he made remarks like "When they're not appreciative to me, they're not appreciative to the Army Corps, they're not appreciative to FEMA, it's not right." These are the people he would unabashedly accuse of the "political weaponization" of the crisis—the very strategy that was his own bread and butter. Politicizing the pandemic was his trademark, it was an expedient and useful cause célèbre to advance his agenda, which was to win re-election.

President Trump started a new round of name-calling by labelling Michigan Governor Gretchen Whitmer "half-Whit" and by using terms like "a snake" and "a nasty person" to describe Washington Governor Jay Inslee—two adjectives that might have occurred to President Trump when he peered into his looking glass while shaving that morning. President Trump had previously ventured an opinion about California Governor Gavin Newsome when he stated in a 2018 rally "How about this clown in California who's running for **governor?**"

The cumulative effect of these lies, hints, and allegations was to cower governors into either accepting the party line or facing a consequential loss of funding. Like Governor Lepetomane in Blazing Saddles, President Trump had to "protect my phony-baloney job," and to do so, governors needed to rubber stamp whatever plan he rolled out, no matter how ludicrous that plan might be or how or dangerous its implementation would prove to be in their respective states. He found many such supplicants when "governors of several of the hardest-hit states sought gingerly Sunday to avoid provoking him anew and risk losing desperately needed federal aid."[16]

On April 30, the President declared that federal social distancing guidelines "will not be extended further" once they ended on May 1. Many governors pushed back on this concept; Illinois' Governor Pritzker extended social distancing until the end of May, then to the end of June, July, August, September, and onward as required.

Pritzker's cautious action and the reluctance of other governors to roll back social distancing guidelines sounded like mutiny to President Trump, and that is exactly what he called it when he tweeted "A good old fashioned mutiny every now and then is an exciting and invigorating thing to watch, especially when the mutineers need so much from the Captain." In that atavistic tweet our President managed to misquote both Thomas Jefferson, who wrote, "I hold it that a little rebellion now and then is a good thing, and as necessary in the political world as storms in the physical," and Captain Marko Ramius, who in The Hunt for Red October observed that "A little revolution now and then is a healthy thing."

President Trump promoted himself from Captain to Monarch when he declared that "when somebody is the president of the United States, the authority is total." Using a strategy that in any other context would constitute a criminal violation of 18 U.S. Code Section 597, which penalizes "Whoever solicits, accepts, or receives any such expenditure in consideration of his vote or the withholding of his vote," President Trump told the nation on May 1 that he would use financial aid to states as his carrot and stick. He would like to help blue states, "but we're going to have to get something for it." The announcement was consistent with his unhitched understanding of electoral fraud, from which quid-pro-quo arrangements he made with Presidents Vladimir Putin and Xi Jinping from 2017 to 2018 were exempted.

The British publication Independent accurately appraised the danger of "threatening to turn federal assistance into leverage for states' compliance" when it stated "Doing so could put at risk some of those who have contracted the Coronavirus, if their local hospital was limited in its ability to treat that person due to a governor's feud with Mr Trump."[17] The Independent stated it would be difficult to force governors "to comply with an order he has yet to even legally justify." Even if President Trump was unaware that his "total authority" declaration was in direct conflict with the Tenth Amendment to the Constitution, the governors being forced to comply certainly had it on their radar.

Carolyn Goodman, the Mayor of Las Vegas, allied herself with President Trump in his war on anyone who expressed unwillingness to comply with re-opening deadlines. On April 21 Goodman was interviewed by MSNBC's Katy Tur. During the interview Goodman hypothesized "Assume everybody is a carrier. And then you start from an even slate. And tell the people what to do. And let the businesses open and competition will destroy that business if, in fact, they (sic) become evident that they have disease, they're closed down. It's that simple." The COVID-19 crisis had not produced many advocates of Social Darwinism; Goodman was the sole owner of that honor. She neglected to point out that when the casinos re-opened prematurely, what happens in Las Vegas would *not* stay in Las Vegas.

The next day, in a twenty-five-minute interview with CNN's Anderson Cooper, Ms. Goodman declined to take the high road and apologize for her idiotic remarks. Instead, she damned the torpedoes and forged ahead, stating in all sincerity, "I'd love everything open, because I think we've had viruses for years that have been here." She quipped "This isn't China, it's Las Vegas." The typically unflappable Cooper "was left exasperated by her comments; at one point, he even covered his face with both hands."[18]

Goodman further suggested that residents of and visitors to Las Vegas would function as both a "control group" and a "placebo" to determine if anyone contracted COVID-19 due to their sty in Sin City. Mr. Cooper realized that it would be a colossal waste of time to define the word "placebo" for her and to tell Mayor Goodman that no one group could simultaneously be an experimental group and a control group. Instead, he reminded the Mayor that an immediate re-opening of her city would turn casinos into "petri dishes." Goodman responded, "You're being an alarmist."

When Ms. Goodman denied that the Coronavirus could be spread in a restaurant, Mr. Cooper advised her twice that her statement was "really ignorant." He found it difficult to keep the discussion on track when he heard non sequiturs like "You're talking about disease. I'm talking about life and living." She dodged his question "Would you feel safe visiting a re-opened casino?" by replying first, that she did not gamble, and second, that the casinos on Las Vegas Boulevard were not controlled by the city of Las Vegas. Anderson Cooper politely thanked her and ended the interview.

The next day Anderson Cooper spoke with Nevada Governor Steve Sisolak, who intellectually and socially-distanced himself from the Mayor, stating "I will not allow the citizens of Nevada, our Nevadans, to be used as a control group, as a placebo, whatever she wants to call it." He assured viewers that before Las Vegas opened, his state would "establish the best protocols for a safe and sustainable re-opening." "We want to welcome everyone back to Las Vegas," he specified, "but that will not be today, and it will not be tomorrow." The date turned out to be June 4, but nonetheless Governor Sisolak reassured his citizens and viewers that "I am not going to put workers in a position where they have to decide between their jobs and their paychecks, and their lives."

The two statements that most put Governor Sisolak at odds with the President's Mayday Re-Opening Celebration were "We can't wait to welcome you—when the time is right" and "I'm listening to the medical people, I'm listening to the scientists...they will decide when it's safe to re-open in a phased-in approach." "Who the hell does he think he is," Mr. Trump must have wondered, "to figure he's the one to determine when the time is right!"

President Trump did not appreciate the Governor's "In your face!" statement that science and data will dictate the timing of a phased-in approach. That was a decision that the President believed he alone should make, since he was Mr. Authority, you know, the person who declared about testing, "No, I don't take responsibility at all because we were given a set of circumstances, and we were given rules, regulations and specifications from a different time."

President Trump had never liked Sisolak, who defeated Trump endorsee Adam Laxalt in that state's 2018 gubernatorial race. Now, two years later, he could show Sisolak who is running this show. Undaunted, the Governor stuck to his guns and announced on April 28 "I am able to make announcements this week because so many of you have stayed home for Nevada and helped flatten the curve against #COVID19...I look forward to this next phase in the battle against COVID-19—one that will be federally supported, state managed, & locally executed."

"With that attitude," President Trump must have decided, "Sisolak will have a better chance of getting money if he goes to a Bellagio roulette table and puts it all on double zero." President Trump knew how to win casino wars—he had bankrupted three of them in Atlantic City: the Taj Mahal, Trump Plaza, and Trump Castle. The President was certain that Mayor Goodman had the right idea, but she lacked the power to make it happen. The President of the United States, on the other hand, owned that power. He would open Las Vegas city and county casinos even if that action meant they would close their doors a month later.

President Trump knew that re-opening the economy would cost lives, but that fact did not alter his course. President Trump expressed the same, regrettable position in July, regarding the re-opening of public schools in September 2020. The CDC had established guidelines for a safe return to school. President Trump stated on July 8 that he "may cut off funding" for schools that did not fully re-open without employing the "very tough" and "expensive" standards of social distancing recommended by the CDC. He brought the same economic carrot and stick to bear when he stated, "We're very much going to put pressure on governors and everybody else to open the schools, to get them open."

Warned that an unsafe re-opening of schools would result in more transmissions and more deaths, President Trump ignored those inevitable consequences and ordered children back to school, an action which would enable parents to return to work, which he felt would lead to a greater economic recovery by election time. Any other President might have said, "The measures to protect the safety of our children and their families when schools re-open will be very tough and expensive, but we will do them anyway, because lives are more important than money." But from 2016 to 2020, we were not blessed with wise leadership.

Consequently, it did not matter to Mr. Trump that children would transmit COVID-19 to their parents who would in turn re-enter the work force to infect other employees, leading to an exponential increase of positive COVID-19 cases. Nor did it bother him one iota that teachers would work in an uncontrolled environment, and they and their families would fall prey to the spiral of infection, hospitalization, and death. He had once again shown that he possessed the mettle to make the wrong, deadly decision if he could profit politically from its outcome.

It is always a difficult decision for any President to order troops to war, knowing that many would not return alive to our soil. Presidents have not condemned civilians to their deaths, yet that is exactly what President Trump did. He possessed an abundance of that immoral willingness. His unbridled lust for getting himself re-elected put Americans in harm's way. He would not wait for "the best protocol for a safe and sustainable re-opening" to materialize. He downplayed civilian risk of life on May 4 by stating "The people of our country should think of themselves as warriors" before he departed for Arizona to visit a Honeywell factory that produced N-95 masks. Six weeks later, Arizona would record the highest rates of COVID-19 infections in our country, topping the number of new cases per day that New York had experienced at the apex of its infections.

When Air Force One landed at Sky Harbor Airport in Phoenix, Mr. Trump emerged from the airplane without wearing a face covering. He exposed Honeywell workers to possible contamination when he and his entourage toured the factory without a mask. CNN's Kevin Liptak wondered if the real purpose was political because "the state is also a critical battleground Trump hopes to win in November's general election. He began an address at the factory by recalling his 2016 election win."[19]

The President's foreknowledge of loss of life due to premature re-opening was apparent when he stated, "Will some people be affected? Yes. Will some people be affected badly? Yes. But we have to get our country open." He made that statement at a time when "many states have re-upped their restrictions and only a few states have seen the prolonged decline in cases the federal government says is necessary before phasing out social distancing."[20]

In the 1959 Lewis Milestone film Pork Chop Hill, when Lt. Joe Clemmons (Gregory Peck) was asked if it was worth fighting for a hill "of no particular strategic military value," he replied, "Nothing's got a value except the value that men put upon it, and I don't know how men can put a higher value on something than dying for it." For President Trump, the act of restarting the economy so he could be re-elected possessed the same value for him as Pork Chop Hill did for Lt. Clemmons. Trump was willing and eager to pay that terrible cost of American lives to ensure himself of a second term.

One important difference between the two situations is that along with the lives of men under his command, Lt. Clemmons risked his own life defending the Korean hill, while President Trump relegated himself to the safer role of a sideline cheerleader. He was like the baseball manager who orders a suicide squeeze play, knowing his runner on third base would be mauled by the catcher defending home plate. President Trump ordered states to re-open when he knew that a premature opening would have the most tragic consequences and would cause the number of positive cases to spike throughout the country. To put it more simply, he *did not care.*

The economy had to be stimulated if he hoped to succeed on November 3, and to do that, he would declare the country safe—that is, safe enough to hold political rallies. President Trump stated on numerous occasions that an inability to hold political rallies "would put me at great disadvantage," but the President's logic was murky because no rallies for him meant no rallies for Joe Biden. President Trump never favored a level playing field.

Trump Administration officials generated models that predicted three thousand more deaths per day in June if guidelines for a "safe and sustainable re-opening" were ignored. Nonetheless, President Trump proceeded full speed ahead, like the eleven Iranian gunboat leaving the scene of the incursion, escaping flares fired from the "AC-130 gunships and Apache attack helicopters" that were used "to defend (our) presence in the Persian Gulf."[21]

After indicting China and the World Health Organization, and after abusing U.S. governors, President Trump targeted President Obama as the person responsible for our lack of pandemic preparedness. When President Trump "was asked by the ultra-sycophantic One America News Network" if he viewed failure to contain the Coronavirus as "a function of lax oversight from the Obama/Biden administration," he replied "We inherited a lot of garbage. We took, ah, they had tests that were no good, they had, all the stuff was no good. It came from somewhere, so whoever came up with it. Our stockpiles were empty. We had horrible stockpiles, we had horrible ventilators, we had very few of them too...CDC had obsolete tests, old tests, broken tests, and a mess."[22] Such a charge is as ridiculous blaming Madame Curie for Little Boy and Fat Man, or cursing Benjamin Franklin because solar energy is not more cost efficient. Perhaps President Trump was unaware that it is not possible to test for a virus that does not exist.

President Trump found precedence and justification for laying such blame at President Obama's feet by harking back to the H1N1 Swine Flu epidemic of 2009 to 2010. Sixty-one million cases of that influenza were reported, causing the death of twelve thousand Americans. To put that figure in perspective, by July 14, 2020, one hundred and thirty-eight thousand Americans people died of COVID-19. President Trump's mismanagement of the Coronavirus pandemic caused eleven times more deaths in less than one-half of the time it took for H1N1 to reach its sad tally.

President Trump had the audacity to tweet on March 13 that President Obama's "response to H1N1 Swine Flu was a full scale disaster, with thousands dying." Since "thousands," meaning twelve thousand, rightfully constituted a "full-scale disaster," what are we to make of eleven or perhaps twenty times that number of deaths? Is any multiple acceptable if it is less than the two hundred thousand deaths President Trump predicted might occur when he addressed the nation in February 2020?

On May 4, The New York Times reported that, due to premature re-opening of the country, "The daily death toll will reach about 3,000 on

June 1, a 70 percent increase from the current number of about 1,750." The Times article also noted that "projections, based on government modeling pulled together by the Federal Emergency Management Agency, forecast about 200,000 new cases each day by the end of the month, up from about 25,000 cases a day currently."[23]

President Trump often used the statement "one death is too many" as a euphemism. For anyone who sincerely believed that one death is too many, the only correct and moral course of action should be to make sure there will not be two deaths. This crucial element prevalent in the psychology of a rational man escaped President Trump's purview. His approach to the pandemic was neither Cartesian nor holistic; it was scattered, self-contradictory, and selfish. His was at best a utilitarian strategist, with his brass ring being re-election. It did not matter to our unmasked President that his denials and blames, his actions and inactions exacerbated the imminently lethal threat that the Coronavirus posed to the health, safety, and lives of thousands of more Americans. At the beginning of May he declared that the situation was "well under control," even though the likelihood of more deaths occurring due to a prematurely re-opened economy was a statistical certainty.

The media has been a convenient and life-long scapegoat for Donald Trump. Throughout the entirety of the Coronavirus Task Force briefings at the White House, President Trump castigated the pool of reporters, calling them nasty and disgraceful and terrible and ultimately fake. When he did not like a question, he told the reporter that he or she was "never going to make it." On March 29 he told PBS reporter Yamiche Alcindor "Come on, come on. Why don't you people—why don't you act in a little more positive? It's always, 'Getcha, getcha, getcha.' And you know what? That's why nobody trusts the media anymore." On April 5 he scolded an AP reporter, stating he should not be asking "wise guy questions," and that the Associated Press was "not like it used to be." He has lambasted the media for being "so unfair" to him, and he has pigeonholed reporters as being "among the most dishonest human beings on Earth."

According to the President reporters should not be "so horrid in the way you ask a question"—he would prefer a format where reporters began each question with "Congratulations" and ended each question with "what a great job, a beautiful job you are doing!" On April 6, President Trump told reporter Francesca Chambers that she was "incapable of asking a question in a positive way."[24] Later in the briefing he told all reporters present "I wish we had a fair media in this country, and we really don't."

To clarify the President words, when he said "in a positive way," by positive he meant "in a groveling way," and when he said "a fair media," he meant media coverage that was lopsided in his favor. Apparently Mr. Trump views himself as a reborn Colonel Nathan R. Jessep who, at the end of A Few Good Men, asserted "I have neither the time nor the inclination to explain myself to a man who rises and sleeps under the blanket of the very freedom that I provide, then questions the manner in which I provide it. I would rather you just said thank you and went on your way." That smugness was a sufficient cause for Jessep's arrest and a prevailing factor in the impeachment of a President.

President Trump displayed a fully dictatorial penchant whenever he addressed the media, but he was equally capable of playing the victim when it suited him. His "poor me" lament reached a pinnacle on May 3 when he conducted a Town Hall Meeting with two Fox interviewers present at the Lincoln Memorial. The event, advertised as "America Together: Returning to Work," provided a perfect venue for Mr. Trump. It permitted him to make a facile comparison between Abraham Lincoln and himself. President Trump stated "They always said Lincoln — nobody got treated worse than Lincoln. I believe I am treated worse."

President Trump described his approach to the pandemic as playing "a very complicated game of chess or poker. Name whatever you want to name. But it's not checkers. That I can tell you. We have a very complicated game going." His was a chilling analogy, because no scientist, doctor, health care worker, first responder, prisoner, nursing home resident, minority group member, elderly person, or anyone sick with COVID-19 viewed the pandemic as a game. His re-opening plans were not predicated on positive results from careful studies or by any objective data. Countless more lives were at stake, and we did not need to hear from him that fighting the pandemic was tougher than winning a game which any eight-year old could master with a little practice. We knew better than President Trump how high were the stakes.

Perhaps President Trump views himself as possessing the skill set required to solve the problem. He has claimed to know more about the Coronavirus than anyone else does. Just as likely though is the interpretation that his statements are no more than common braggadocio. Either way, none of us who viewed that Town Hall event had learned anything new. We were no better equipped to understand our nation's response to the pandemic at the conclusion of the Town Hall than we were at the beginning of the program. Instead of facts, we received empty reassurances. Instead of hearing sincere words sympathy we received glad-hand platitudes from President Trump. Instead of being led to appreciate that every life matters and being told that no steps would be taken that would increase the likelihood of more deaths, we were mollycoddled into believing that more deaths were a low price to pay for economic rebirth. If we named the game President Trump was playing that night, it was not be checkers—it was three-card monte. We were once more deceived by the con man who stole an election four years ago, the one who swore to preserve, protect, and defend our Constitutional rights.

The firing and discrediting of public officials who disagreed with President Trump was another tool he used to deflect blame for the increase of cases of infections and deaths. Rick Bright and Tony Fauci are two such examples.

Dr. Rick Bright had served as the Deputy Assistant Secretary with the Department of Health and Human Services, and he led our Biomedical Advanced Research and Development Agency (BARDA). He was exactly the right man in the right place at the right time to guide the nation through the crisis of a pandemic.

An expert in vaccines, Dr. Bright reported to Dr. Robert Kadlec, a Republican who served the President as Assistant Secretary for Preparedness and Response at the Department of Health and Human Services. Kadlec's supervisor was Health and Human Services Secretary Alex Azar.

Dr. Bright ran afoul of Kadlec as early as 2018 when he objected to "the outsized role Dr. Kadlec allowed industry consultants to play in securing contracts that Dr. Bright and other scientists and subject matter experts determined were not meritorious." In January 2020 Dr. Bright warned his supervisor that we should expect to encounter a Coronavirus pandemic "but he encountered opposition from Trump administration officials" and consequently he "was transferred out of BARDA in retaliation."

On April 20 Dr. Bright "was transferred to a 'less impactful position' at the National Institute of Health after he was reluctant to promote the use of drugs such as hydroxychloroquine to treat COVID-19 patients." In a whistleblower complaint filed by Dr. Bright, he "objected to these efforts and made (it) clear that BARDA would only invest the billions of dollars allocated by Congress to address the COVID-19 pandemic in safe and scientifically vetted solutions and it would not succumb to the pressure of politics or cronyism."[25]

Because Dr. Bright was not the yes-man that Kadlec, Azar, and President Trump had hoped he would be, he was fired. Mind-boggling as it seems, a renowned expert in vaccines and epidemics was dismissed for political reasons, not for any failure to perform adequately at a high-level position. Again, the American people would pay the price for keeping the President's men in line.

President Trump was not pleased by a statement made by Dr. Anthony Fauci on May 26, when Fauci testified to Congress that we could avoid a second wave of COVID-19, that a resurgence could be limited in tis impact *if* states "re-opened in a smart way." The President figured that sooner or later, someone was going to pay for throwing a monkey wrench into the works—maybe Anthony Fauci.

When a poll indicated that twice as many Americans found Dr. Fauci to be more a more credible source of information than President Trump, the White House choreographed a plan to discredit Dr. Fauci, who had already been excluded from Task Force briefings and press conference appearances. On July 13 President Trump called Fauci "Dr. Gloom and Doom," and stated that the Doctor "is a very nice man, but he's made a lot of mistakes." A White House memo alleged that officials "are concerned about the number of times Dr. Fauci has been wrong on things."

At the top of that list of officials is Admiral Brett Giroir who, as our "testing czar" said Dr. Fauci is "not 100 percent right" because he wanted to shut down states which experienced post-Fourth of July COVID-19 surges, and because Fauci has "a very narrow public health point of view."

Viewing the pandemic from a public health, not a political point of view was in the best interest of Americans, but it did not serve the minacious interests of the President. Dr. Fauci was given the boot as quickly and expeditiously as Dr. Bright.

Politics informed President Trump's decision to remove Intelligence Community Inspector General Michael Atkinson, after Atkinson notified Congress of the events leading to the Ukraine scandal and ultimately to the President's impeachment. The swift dismissal of Atkinson empowered President Trump to remove Acting Department of Defense Inspector General Glenn Fine. Fine had been serving as the chairperson of the Pandemic Response Accountability Committee.

The President did not trust Fine, who" had a reputation as a bulldog investigator" to "monitor government spending under the new $2 trillion relief bill,"[26] so the President replaced him with Sean O'Donnell before nominating Jason Abend, a friend of his who had served as a policy advisor at Customs and Border Control, to replace O'Donnell. Abend would play ball with President Trump. The fact that Abend had "no experience running a large organization, unlike many previous Pentagon IG's, and no military background"[27] was not a substantive drawback in the eyes of the President.

By firing Fine for "incompetence" and alleging that his shortcomings made the battle against the Unseen Enemy more difficult, our Teflon President solidified his power base over the dispersal of C.A.R.E.S. funds. The President's actions followed a well-defined pattern. He dismissed reporters' accusations as "media hype," when he himself was the original hypester. He blamed the previous Administration which he alleged had failed to prepare adequately for this pandemic. According to President Trump, President Obama had installed incompetent appointees and derelict Inspectors General.

The hypocrisy of that accusation was borne out when, along with Inspectors General Atkinson and Fine, he fired for political reasons—not for due cause—Inspector General Mitch Behm from the Department of Transportation, Inspector General Christi Grimm for Health and Human Services, and Inspector General Steve Linick from the State Department. Geoffrey Berman, the U.S. Attorney for the Southern District of New

York paid the price for the President's shortcomings on June 20, when he was fired by the Chief Executive.

President Trump blamed the greedy, ignorant, and insolent governors of New York, California, New Jersey, and other blue states for causing hotspots in their respective domains. He blamed The World Health Organization for allegedly befriending China and consequently mishandling the pandemic, stating "By the time you finally declared the virus a pandemic on March 11,2020, it had killed more than 4,000 people and infected more than 100,000 people in at least 114 countries around the world." He did not mention that by March 11, due to his own mishandling of the pandemic, President Trump could claim the credit for twenty-five percent of the four thousand deaths he alleged were caused by the World Health Organization.

He blamed China for the high number of cases in the United States, for the rapid spread of the Coronavirus in the United States, and for COVID-19 deaths in the United States, all of which could have been minimized had our President acted on information he had received in January 2020.

When President Trump's dislike of how Doctors Fauci and Brix failure to support his pie-in-the-sky prognoses reached critical mass, he ended the daily televised Coronavirus Task Force Briefings. As if the end of the briefings wasn't bad enough news for Americans searching for answers and getting none from the President, on May 5 President Trump announced he was "winding down" his Coronavirus Task Force, echoing Vice President Pence's remarks that the Task Force would be "dismantled." The next day the President seemed to reverse that position, stating that the present Task Force would change—it would be augmented and "re-focused," and he would "add or subtract people to it, as appropriate." President Trump would find boon compatriots more willing to stand in his shadow and to swear that taking hydroxychloroquine was an effective COVID-19 remedy.

On May 6, Press Secretary Kayleigh McEnany whimsically responded to a question about testing. Jim Acosta asked, "Shouldn't all Americans who go back to work be able to get a test before they do, to feel comfortable in their own work environment to be interacting with other individuals?" Her reply encapsulated the condescension and effrontery the

Administration feels toward the American public. She could have reasonably replied to that soft ball question by saying, "yes, that's what we hope governors and employers will insist upon."

Instead, Ms. McEnany had the audacity to imply that you can never satisfy any one—that if you give one person a test, pretty soon everyone is going to want a test, and after they got one, they would want another one, cycling in an ever-widening gyre. That was precisely what she did say when she answered, "Let's dismiss a myth about tests right now. If we tested every single American in this country at this moment, we'd have to retest them an hour later and then an hour later after that. Because, at any moment you could theoretically contract this virus. So the notion that everyone needs to be tested is just simply nonsensical."[28]

By stating the above, she castigated the American public for its insatiable and child-like self-centeredness, and she blamed the average American employee for not understanding of how safely and simply a return to work order could be accomplished. According to Ms. McEnany, American workers were never content, and now they wanted to complicate President Trump's best laid plan by bringing up issues of health and tests. She might have well have asked, "Why couldn't they leave well-enough alone and go back to sweeping floors in nursing homes, walking the night shift at Tehachapi, and cutting sides of beef into steaks at the JBS plant in Moore County, Texas?"

Her reply constituted yet another case of a Presidential syndrome better known as "Who are you going to believe, me or your lying eyes?" When President Trump eventually fires McEnany for some real or perceived indiscretion, with her demonstrated and facile ability to reassure us that we should *not* worry about COVID-19 infection when we return to our non-socially-distanced jobs, Kayleigh McEnany won't have much trouble finding new employment. In fact, she could win the starring role in a new Twilight Zone episode entitled "Sleep Well, Kids, Because There's No Bloodthirsty Monster Hiding Under Your Beds."

When she was asked about our relationship with China, Ms. McEnany re-stated the President's default position of blaming China for his own failure to act quickly and decisively to contain the Coronavirus. She summarized that attitude by explaining, "Right now it is a relationship of disappointment and frustration. The President has said how frustrated he is at some of the decisions of China that put American lives at risk."

I would speculate that President Trump does not have any idea of the apotheosis of disappointment and frustration that we feel because of his mishandling of the Coronavirus pandemic. On May 7 actor Robert De Niro told Stephen Colbert on A Late Show that he was "at a loss of words" to describe his disappointment with the inactions of the current Administration, which has resulted in so many deaths. Like the rest of us, Mr. De Niro was at a loss to understand President Trump's callous statement of May 6, when President Trump asseverated that "Americans may have to accept that re-opening will cause more deaths."

By the end of the first week of May, we shared Mr. De Niro's inability to describe our vexatious sense of disappointment in our government's approach to the pandemic. Our fear of dying from COVID-19 was an easier but far more frightening and painful perspective to articulate.

Chapter Four

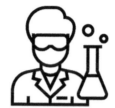

Testing and Measurements

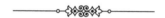

Before I went to sleep at 6 p.m. on the evening of March 30 I set the clock alarm on my phone to chime at 3 a.m. My goal was to arrive at the test site by 4 a.m. and be one of the first one hundred and fifty people to receive a COVID-19 test the next morning. I had heard on the news that by 10 a.m. on the 30th the supply had been exhausted, and that by 7a.m. the line was a half-mile long. I was sure that health care workers, first responders, and anyone in the Chicagoland area with political connections would be in a separate, shorter line, and those people might consume up to a hundred of the two hundred and fifty precious tests allotted by the federal government to be performed on any given day. I did not want to end up holding the bag, being the two hundred and fifty-first customer.

To eliminate experiencing that extreme disappointment, I figured a 4 a.m. arrival would be required. I was aware that testing would most likely continue throughout the week, but there was no guarantee that the drive-in site would not close as quickly as it had materialized, due to a lack of tests. Perhaps the daily test allotment later in the week would decrease. I could not be sure that a riot would not occur when people who had been in line for many hours found out the supply of tests was exhausted. Maybe each car in line ahead of me would contain multiple passengers to be tested. I did not want to leave a matter of this importance to chance. My attempt to get a test had been previously foiled by bureaucracy and I would not allow that to happen to me again.

These worries occupied my thoughts as I tried to fall asleep at the ridiculous hour of 6 p.m. Over the past few days, I had been so tired that I routinely slept between twelve and fourteen hours each night. It was never a sound sleep; I was awakened every two hours by bad dreams and coughing jags and night sweats and shooting pains in my joints and chest. I could not understand why I did not have much of an appetite until I noticed that my sense of taste had been substantially diminished by the infection from which I was suffering. Since I could not taste much of anything, it made sense that I would not care to eat much food or very often.

The only primary taste receptor that seemed to be working provided me with an ability to recognize anything that tasted salty. Food had to be either savory or incredibly spicy for me to notice its presence. Each time I over-flavored my food in this manner I felt like I had turned into the Observer named September in the J.J. Abrams science fiction television series Fringe. September had come to our world from a different timeline in parallel universe. In a scene in Episode Four of Season One, September ordered a beef sandwich at a diner. Because his taste buds were not accustomed to our food, he added two ounces of ground black pepper, eleven jalapenos, and a half-bottle of hot sauce so that his meal would have a noticeable flavor.

My sense of smell did not fare any better. When I saw smoke rising from the top of my toaster, I knew that I had set its level of heat intensity too high. When I checked the digital display, I saw that it registered eight on a scale of ten. It should have been set on a safer, golden-brown level of four. It did not bother me that I had somehow jostled the knob, pushing it toward the high end. The part I found worrisome is that if I had not seen smoke rising, the only way I would have been away of toast burning would have been when it set off my smoke alarm. To my genuine surprise, I noticed that my sense of smell had slowly deteriorated over the weeks until it had all but disappeared. My first impulse was that the olfactory change was due to my general stuffiness, but upon reflection, I noticed that during the rare times when I could breathe more easily, I still could not detect the citrus scent in a bar of verbena soap, the alcohol scent in an open bottle of Crown Royal, or the eucalyptus scent in the cough drops I had been consuming by the handful.

I looked online to see if loss of these two senses had been reported by other COVID-19 patients. Try as I might, I could not find any information about a loss of the ability to taste food or detect scents. The absence of data did not surprise me, because other than reports of general symptoms like coughing, sneezing, headaches, and temperatures, there was no information to be had about any specific symptoms that tens of thousands of COVID-19 were encountering. I had begun to wonder how long the headache or temperature components of the disease would last, but lack of information foiled my line of inquiry.

I hoped I was not alone in experiencing what I regarded as weird symptoms, because that recognition would be disconcerting. With no apparent standard of measurement available, I assumed very unscientifically that my symptoms were typical and not worth another moment of worry. The best solution that occurred to me was to scale down the toaster temperature and not open that bottle of Crown Royal, which each evening beckoned to me from my cabinet like sirens of Titan summoning Winston Niles Rumfoord to his destiny.

I recall not sleeping much that night. I was used to the caffeine present in the aspirin I was taking to control my temperature, so that was not the cause. Anxiety and trepidation about what would happen the next morning were the culprits. At 8 p.m. I realized that I had no way of knowing if my car would start on the morning that I most needed it to function properly. I had not been away from home for nearly two weeks. I would need to visit a grocery store soon to replenish my supply of pasta, olive out, and vegetables, and March 30 would have been a good day to accomplish those errands and to have my car checked by a Toyota mechanic, but all those ideas had slipped my mind. My upcoming test occupied the entirety of my cerebral cortex.

I had gone to bed before the weather report segment of the evening news had aired. The outside temperature in the early morning would most likely be in the high twenties. The very thought made me shiver. At 8 p.m. I got out of bed and set a blanket, a warm hat, gloves, a small pillow, and my

Edie Bauer down parka on my kitchen table. At 10 p.m. I was thirsty and went for a drink of water, but when I got to the kitchen I realized that if I arrived at the test site by 330 a.m. and testing did not start until 9 a.m. in a best case scenario, I would be in my car for seven hours with no access to a restroom, so I went back to bed without drinking anything.

I tried to get comfortable for an hour until I climbed out of bed and stumbled in the dark until I found where I had stashed a new box of Kleenex. My seemingly random actions late at night provided quality entertainment for Sonia. She usually sleeps on a blanket at the foot of my bed, and my guess was that she wondered why I kept disturbing her slumber.

Midnight seemed to be a reasonable time to verify that my Illinois Driver's License was still in my wallet. I was fully engaged in senseless and obsessive behaviors which were counterproductive to the goal of somnolence, but I was not able to stop myself. I wondered if President Trump was madly tweeting or resting comfortably. It must be nice, I thought, to have not a care in the world other than to determine how best to use social media to insult someone whom I felt had done me wrong.

At 130 a.m. I was in a hypnagogic state, imagining a line longer than the one I encountered at the Department of Motor Vehicles each time I went for a vision test. I was sure my mindset was the same as the attitude held by everyone else planning to arrive for an early morning test. I wondered what would happen, once I arrived at the testing site as planned, when it was my turn to proceed. Would my car fail to start at that crucial juncture? If that happened, once I put the gear in neutral, would I have enough energy to push the car the rest of the way, and call AAA after the test was completed? Is that what my life had come to at age sixty-nine?

It was a sobering thought, one which led me to question if my car had sufficient fuel to idle for six hours. At 145 a.m. I contemplated going outside and checking my car's fuel supply, but I thought better of that plan, because if I stepped foot outside of my condo now, too many things could go wrong. What if I dropped my keys down the sewer? What if I locked the car with the keys inside? Perhaps fate would allow the car to start only once that morning, and I would have squandered that opportunity by needlessly powering it up to check on the fuel supply.

At 2 a.m. I needed a reality check. There was no one I could call at that hour to whom I could rant senselessly about what bad timing it would be if a global extinction event occurred before I got tested. Although I couldn't take deep breaths to relax, I could remain motionless and think only pleasant thoughts, like how nice it will be in a few short months to go to Oak Street Beach to get a tan, but mostly to admire the latest trends in women's beachwear, taking note of the fine and minimalist fashions on display at Chicago's hottest beach.

Perhaps on that a sun-kissed day President Trump would call Jared Kushner an idiot and would apologize to Nancy Pelosi and Andrew Cuomo but mostly to the American public, and to prove the sincerity of his expression of regret, he would hand over control of the Coronavirus pandemic to the scientists and doctors, to the CDC, and to the NIH. To make further amends to the American people, President Trump would declare a general amnesty on paying any 2019 and 2020 federal income tax for everyone whose livelihood had been negatively affected by the way he mishandled the crisis. Those were the comforting misconceptions that lulled me to sleep that night, approximately a half-hour before my cell phone sounded its alarm.

I thought "You've got to be kidding," and I was about to roll over to sleep for another few minutes when I came to my senses. I recalled the acoustic opening of Supertramp's "Give a Little Bit," when Roger Hodgson sang, "Alright, here we go again." His words provided the exhortation I needed. As I washed my face, I felt calm. My anxiety was temporarily reduced, replaced by a sense of relief that this was finally happening. Before long I would be back in bed getting some sleep, happy that my test had been completed.

I had spent hours that night rehearsing in my head what would happen when I awoke, and I followed my mental check list. I dressed and made sure my phone, wallet, and keys were securely located on my person. I donned my parka, grabbed a carryon bag which now held my blanket, pillow, hat, and gloves, and exited, remembering to lock the door. I climbed into my car which started on the first try. I left my parking spot and drove on a deserted Northwest Highway to Harlem Avenue. I knew exactly where I was going. I had been to the test site many times a decade ago to have my car's emission level checked. Barring the occurrence of any bizarre car accident, of any other baroque or preternatural circumstance, in twenty minutes I would be parked in line on Forest Preserve Drive.

When I arrived at 3:45 a.m. I wondered if I was indeed in the right place because there was no long line of cars. As closely as I could determine, I was the fourth car in line! It was a bit hard to see further ahead because a large, white Cadillac Escalade had secured the spot in front of me. I could see a woman's face for a moment when she turned on the cabin's interior lights and leaned to the side of her headrest to light her cigarette while she talked on her cell phone.

I wondered how she could smoke and talk while I could not talk without coughing. Perhaps her symptoms were not as severe as mine. Maybe she would test negative. If she tested positive, maybe that finding would convince her to stop smoking, but if she were a nicotine addict, that outcome was unlikely. I worried that she would get cancer, resulting in her talking on her phone through a voice box like the character named Gray Baker that Andy Garcia portrayed in Kenneth Branagh's 1991 film <u>Dead Again</u>.

I had never smoked cigarettes. I found it counterproductive to my habit of running long distances, although I admit cigarette smoking did not stop Lord Andrew Lindsay from winning a silver medal in the four-hundred meter hurdles event in the 1924 Paris Summer Olympics. I did not think Ms. Escalade was a world class athlete because she surely would have earned a place in the short line at the Testing Site. Perhaps I was wrong, and she would be a hurdles competitor in the upcoming Tokyo Summer Olympics, which were postponed until 2021 on March 21 due to the global pandemic.

I had an excellent view of the Escalade's license plate number; I had several hours to memorize it for no good reason. Our cars were parked adjacent to a fenced off and well-barricaded entrance to the site. To my right I could see the facility. Its outward appearance had not changed. It was approximately a hundred feet wide, forty feet long, and twenty feet tall. It resembled a carport where you could park a semi-tractor trailer in each of its three entrances. It was deserted at that hour. To my left was the large parking lot of an apartment complex.

I turned off my engine, wrapped myself in my blanket, and rested my head against the door window on the pillow I had brought. Five minutes later the blinding Xenon headlights of a blue Nissan sedan parking behind me illuminated more of my car than I needed to see at that moment. Once the those bastardly-bright headlights were dimmed, I watched in my rear-view mirror as a late model Camaro pulled up alongside the Nissan and waited while the Nissan's driver exited his car and entered the Camaro, which then drove away.

A few moments later I realized that the Camaro was the getaway car for Mr. Nissan who wanted his place in line retained by correctly positioning an empty car in line, while he and his co-conspiring spouse went home or to the Motel 6 in Schiller Park to catch another forty winks. I tended to question the ethics of that strategy. Perhaps it was an adaptation of the Chicago philosophy that if you shoveled the snow out of a parking spot in front of your house, no one else should park there. The Nissan was the equivalent of the chairs the homeowner would place in the street to make sure the spot remained inviolate.

In this case, there was no requirement stating that you had to remain in your car while in line, but that was the common-sense assumption. I wondered how he would know what when to return to his car to be sure it moved along with the rest of the line. Had Mr. Nissan developed video capability within his car to monitor the progress? If so, he should be complimented for his forethought and inventiveness, not begrudged for bending the rules of etiquette.

I came to understand very quickly that morning and on a on a deeply personal level the motivation that led to Mr. Nissan to arrive at his efficacious solution. I had driven my Corolla on long trips, but I never sat for what seemed to be an eternity in the driver's seat not going anywhere, without making the movements associated with driving. I had thought I would be comfortable with the seat reclined, but my height made such comfort difficult to attain. There was no place to put my feet if I stretched my legs. The back seat was not wide enough to accommodate a reclined body, and it was getting cold.

I had dressed warmly but I was still breathing air at less than half room temperature, which quickly led to more coughing. I thought it would be amusingly ironic if I contracted pneumonia—if I did not already have it—while waiting to be tested. The only solution for my predicament was to completely cover my head with my blanket, which I was hesitant to do, because I would not know when to move forward if the line began to advance, putting me in the same position as the absent Mr. Nissan.

I was reluctant to idle my car so the heater would work because every time I looked to my right I saw the emission testing site, which reminded me that we all had to do our part to protect the environment, and it would be irresponsibly sinful to release five hours' worth of carbon monoxide into the atmosphere. Ms. Escalade had no such qualms. She was staying warm no matter how badly her CO damaged the atmosphere. I was glad I had parked about a car length behind her; otherwise I would have been breathing enough carbon monoxide to put me to sleep, and I would never again worry about being tested for COVID-19.

I decided to fight the good fight and stay awake, but by 5 a.m. I was prepared to ask Ms. Escalade if I could relax on the second row of seats in her boxy but luxuriously warm and roomy SUV. If she refused me that modest hospitality, I was prepared to lay down in the street, close enough to the Escalade to be warmed by its steady plume of exhaust.

I contented myself with crossing my legs for the hundredth time and listening to my cold, raspy breathing. I would have liked to have played some of the cd's I had brought to pass the time, but it was so cold outside I thought that by doing so, I would use up too much battery power and I would be unable to start the car when it needed to move forward. I figured the car battery was like the battery in my cell phone which expends more power in cold weather. I would never forgive myself if my car would not start because I had listened to my box set of Tom Petty's Live Anthology.

At 530 a.m. I had grown weary of repeating in my head Petty song lyrics like "the waiting is the hardest part." I thought about his song "Out in the Cold" from Into the Great Wide Open, but the foreboding title of that track did not help matters. The lyrics "When I woke up my brain was stunned, I could not come around" warned me of what was likely to happen if I fell asleep, but I was too drowsy to care. I decided to pull my blanket up over my head and grab a few moments of shuteye. I figured a power nap would suit my needs.

When I awoke, an hour had passed and, to my befuddlement, Ms. Escalade was gone. When my glazed-over eyes refocused, I could see a white car of some sort in the distance, far beyond where it had been parked. I panicked because I did not know what had happened. Mr. Nissan was not there to keep a watchful eye and to blow his horn to alert me to move ahead. I wondered if the drivers in front of me had been advised to move forward one by one, and my turn to advance would be soon coming. About a block ahead of me I could see the flashing blue lightbar of a Chicago Police car, but the car was stationary.

It occurred to me that the first car in line may have parked at what appeared to be the entrance to the facility, when the real entrance was further down the road. There was a sign that said "Testing Site" with an arrow that seemed to point at the barricaded entrance near where I had parked, but maybe that sign had been misplaced. Perhaps there were more signs with similar arrows directing customers to move further down the line.

While I was sorting out what to do next, I noticed that the previously unoccupied empty parking lot to my left was now filled with State Police cruisers, and the flashing lights of each car were on full display. Next to those patrol cars was a line of civilian cars, and that line was pointed at the still-barricaded entrance twenty feet in front of me, to my right. I decided to wait a bit, figuring that the Official in Charge of Keeping the Line Moving in an Orderly Fashion had also taken a nap and would soon be back on duty.

I was so transfixed by the State Police cars' flashing lights that I did not notice a black Thunderbird with a single flashing dome light approaching me from the opposite line of traffic. As his car slowed, I rolled down my window. The driver waved to direct me to move ahead and I gave him a thumbs-up sign. I wiped away the fog from my windshield and turned my key in the ignition. I was never so glad to hear that engine start; I had reaped a generous reward for the hours I spent fidgeting during my silent and cold hours of Toyota imprisonment.

After I advanced two blocks, I was certain that my humble place in the history of Community Testing was assured. Being fourth in line guaranteed that in a few hours I would be tested. The hardest part was nearly over.

Though in general I refrain from engaging in lines of thought that would clinically be described as delusional, my lack of sleep had combined with my other symptoms to produce fugue state. When I saw that I had parked my car across from a street sign that read "St. Louis Avenue" I was convinced that I was now playing a roguish part in some bizarre Monopoly game. I envisioned my Corolla to be the racing car token. The back of the SUV parked in front of me resembled the icon in the "Free Parking" game space.

I imagined that I had fallen into an alternate universe, and an evil twin Escalade was now parked in front of me. My consternation was allayed when I saw that the license plate number of the evil twin matched the license plate number that I had memorized so many hours ago. My hands, arms, and legs had gone nearly numb from being in the same position for so long, but the sight of the familiar plate number and the flickering of a lit cigarette in the first dim light of dawn enabled me to maintain an even strain.

At 615 a.m. I heard first one, then several helicopters landing somewhere near a test facility which I could no longer see. I noticed that a <u>WGN</u>-TV News camera truck was stationed to my left, with its microwave antenna raised to a height of about thirty feet. I hoped the helicopters would see the antenna and not hit it in the near-dark. Such a cataclysmic event would certainly delay the day's testing. I realized that the truck was most likely the same one I had seen on television a day before, and since the helicopters were probably flying the same route they had utilized on the 30th, I concluded that the pilots were aware of the obstacle that the elevated antenna posed.

More activity occurred in the next ninety minutes than I had witnessed in the previous hours. The black Thunderbird had once more entered the scene; this time he stopped at each of the three cars in front of me for less than a minute. I was eager to talk to anyone and I rolled down my window once more. The plainclothes officer asked me my age and if I had "Any symptoms?" I told him I was sixty-nine and I had a fever and a cough. With my driver's license in hand, I was prepared to cough or sneeze if requested, but no forms of proof were required.

Satisfied with my reply, the plainclothes officer proceeded on his journey. His next customer should have been Mr. Nissan, but a minute later the driver of a red pickup truck was parking behind me, soon followed by a parade of other cars that were detouring around the Nissan to advance in line. Mr. Nissan's video early warning monitoring system must have failed to alert him to the fact that the time was now, and he was late to the game.

The Chicago Police car with the flashing blue lights was parked where it had been, blocking what I could clearly determine to be the correct driveway entrance to the site. The officer was aligning red traffic cones to form a single lane, through which our cars would pass before doubling back to the test site via an interior access road. I watched as two soldiers in Army camo exited the Chicago Transit Authority Route 78 bus and entered the site through the red-coned lane.

I could hear but could not see more helicopters arriving and departing; I assumed they were delivering the day's ration of tests and supplies. So far everything seemed very well organized, apart from the little snafu about where the line should start. I hoped that the next day would bring more signs or smarter drivers to Forest Preserve Drive, a road which neatly avoided traipsing through an actual Chicago Forest Preserve.

My anticipation turned to eagerness at 7 a.m. when I saw two ladies dressed in the full array of personal protective equipment. Their blue gowns billowed in the morning breeze. Their N-95 face masks, face shields, and goggles minimized the odds of them being infected with COVID-19. Their array also shielded them from a light rain which had begun to fall. With my driver's license still in my hand, I awaited my turn to be interviewed. The tests were not supposed to start until two hours later, but this was a good sign that maybe we would be tested ahead of the publicized schedule.

Both ladies carried clipboards and plastic bags. The first lady asked to see my i.d., and the second one gave me two yellow post-it notes. She had written the number **1** on the first post-it and told me place it on my dashboard along with my photo i.d. I was instructed to write my telephone number on the second and attach it to the inside of my driver's window. I accomplished both of the easy tasks in a minute, placing the number **1** post-it and my driver's license on the left dashboard corner, and writing my phone number backward for ease of reading from the outside before attaching it to my window. I was delighted by the interaction. I believed that it boded well for how simple, quick, and painless the entire operation would be.

Confident that my previous worries were for naught, I congratulated myself on a job well done. I had put in the long hours and the done the hard work. I had gotten myself to a place where I could be tested for COVID-19. I would let the very capable hands of the United States Army guide me to the finish line. I understood the joy and relief that Colonel Nicholson felt when he saw with pride that his bridge on the River Kwai had been completed, and in the nick of time. I judged the unpleasant outcome which befell the Colonel as he watched his world collapse to be an unfortunate aberration, and not something that would in any way apply to me.

I watched in my rearview mirror as the State Police cruisers exited the parking lot where they had been stationed and cordoned off a line of traffic aimed at the previously barricaded test site entrance where I had been parked. I saw each of the civilian cars from the parking lot being directed across the street and into the test site through the entrance that was no longer barricaded. When the cars had completed their migration, someone closed the fifteen-foot-tall iron gates and blocked the driveway with yellow sawhorses.

I had mixed feelings about the Easy Street access the drivers of those cars had been granted. This was a signal that testing was really happening, which was a good thing. Ambivalence surfaced because I wondered how the person far behind me whose place in line had earned him or her the two hundred and fiftieth test would feel had he or she been aware of the line-cutter who had usurped that last remaining test. On the other hand, assuming that those who had been granted this ease of access were health care workers and first responders and their families, then this was by and large the correct procedure to follow. Those people in the short line had earned the right to get back to their jobs and loved ones as quickly as possible. You could not ask EMTs, for example, to wait in a mile-long line when their time would be better utilized caring for the sick. However, because this entire operation was happening within Chicago city limits, that parking lot could have very well been jammed with fortunate sons, like the wife of the cousin of an alderman from a wealthy Chicago ward.

I chose to trust that decency had prevailed, and the people being tested first were the ones risking their lives each day and twice on Sundays to help Coronavirus victims.

I ended my ruminations on whether what was happened behind me was encouraging or depressing and I concentrated on Advancing to Go. The Escalade was directed to move forward, and I was signaled to follow in step. As I made a right turn into the traffic cone lane, I was told to stop. A pfc gave me two multi-colored leaflets. The Escalade had stopped, which gave me time to peruse each handout.

The first page, issued by the U.S. Public Health Services office, was entitled "**Coronavirus COVID 19: WHAT TO EXPECT AT COMMUNITY-BASED SITES.**" Toward the top of the page were two blue blocks. The block to the left contained instructions that might have been helpful to have had on hand *before* arriving at the site. For example, it said, "You must arrive in a personal vehicle." I had nailed that item. Then in bullet points were listed the following requirements:

- **Items to bring:**

  — Photo I.D.

  — Health insurance card (everyone will be tested regardless if they have insurance)

  — Healthcare facility employee or first responder ID/Badge (if applicable)

Based on these criteria, I was All Systems Go.

The blue block to the right was entitled "**THINGS TO CONSIDER.**" Of the five items which followed, the first and last were two of which I had prior knowledge:

- There are **no** bathrooms;

- There may be **significant wait times.**

In between those two immutable and highly significant laws of nature were listed the following instructions:

- Each person who needs testing must be seated next to a **working window**;

- All passengers must **stay inside** vehicles from arrival to departure;

- Try to **limit** the people inside your vehicle to those needing testing

The brochure went on to explain that upon arrival, "Each vehicle will be greeted and directed by personnel in full medical gear." The drivers were being greeted, not the cars, but why quibble, I thought, about such a small syntactical error.

Under the topic of "**TEMPERATURE CHECK**" were the words "Your temperature will be checked using a no touch thermometer." I was quite certain that no one had checked my or my vehicle's temperature.

"**ITEMS TO BRING**" information was reprinted below the blue box, underneath the temperature advisement, under the heading of **REGISTRATION**. After being told we would be asked to provide a photo i.d, we now learned that our i.d. must include a first and last name. I did not worry that this new stipulation would slow down the proceedings at my site, because people with one name like Seal, Cher, Madonna, Bjork, Adele, Ludicrous, or Morrissey probably would not be waiting in this line at Forest Preserve Drive on this date.

A "current address" was required, and to explain things to anyone who did not know the definition of "current address," a parenthetical clarification "(where you are staying)" had been added. I was sure this would cause confusion for anyone currently staying at the Holiday Inn in Bolingbrook but residing in Coeur d'Alene.

The last item to bring was the "Best phone number to reach you (indicate mobile/landline.)" We were not told to specify mobile or landline when we jotted down our phone number on the yellow post-it on the window. I was not sure if I should remove the post-it and scribble "mobile" underneath my phone number. That seemed too risky an action to undertake.

An official could spot the momentarily missing post-it and tell me "Why didn't you put your post-it note on the window like you were supposed to? Go to the end of the line!"

The middle section of the first leaflet addressed the crux of the matter. It was labeled "**TESTING**." The three bullet points under **TESTING** were not complicated, but I had observed in life that bad outcomes occur when simple instructions are not followed. It was easy for example to help yourself to a mountainous slathering of tepid, soft serve ice cream at the Golden Corral buffet and ignore the small cue card which stated, "One Four Ounce Serving Per Customer." The bad outcome involved troublesome gastrointestinal activities two hours later.

The **TESTING** bullet points read:

- A healthcare provider in personal protective equipment will provide you with instructions.

- You will be given a tissue to blow your nose and will need to keep the tissue to dispose on your own.

- A soft swab will be inserted deep into your nose to get the necessary sample. This **may be slightly uncomfortable**; however, the test is quick and should take less than a minute.

Since the first point said that someone would provide instructions, I assumed that those oral, step by step explanations would be sufficient to guide me through this uncharted territory. I should not have taken that sober instruction so seriously, but logic dictated that I should absorb its content and that of the remaining two points, especially number three. The qualification "**may be slightly uncomfortable**" sounded like famous last words, reminding me of how guitarist Terry Kath pointed to the pistol he was holding and said, "Don't worry, it's not loaded."

The last section was more to my liking; it was called "**INFORMATION AND DEPARTURE**." Its bullet points were clear and concise:

- **Once the test is complete, you will move to the final station.**

- You will be given information to take with you on what to do while awaiting your results. **Please keep the instruction sheet until you get your test results.**

- Depart/exit Community Testing Site.

- Follow the instructions on the paper provided by the community-based Testing Site. Continue to monitor and record symptoms. You will receive test results via telephone call.

This was more good news, I thought. The test would soon be over, and I would have my choice of departing or exiting. I would remember not to be a smart aleck and cause trouble by questioning the relative difference between the two terms.

That leaflet ended with a one-line, half-inch wide, navy blue banner which ran across the bottom margin. Its chilling message was already familiar to me, courtesy of the Illinois Department of Public Health. The fine-print banner read "**For Medical Emergencies, call 911 and notify the dispatcher that you may have COVID-19.**"

That final instruction would be easy to follow, but its implication was unnerving. It asserted that my case of COVID-19 could end up placing me in an ambulance going to the nearest hospital that was accepting COVID-19 patients. It was an eventuality that I hoped to avoid, one that I had seen recurring in Washington, California, and New York. Seeing it on a piece of paper I was holding in my hand, though, brought a terrifying sense of immediacy and personal danger into focus. This was a life-threatening event and it was not happening to an obscure subset of unlucky people outside of my frame of reference. It was happening to me. That banner provided a formidable wake up call, one that I could not ignore or silence by hitting a snooze button. In other words, I could not afford to think like Donald Trump.

The second leaflet provided instructions for what I should do after I had been tested. I figured I could read that later, and besides, it was now my turn to inch closer to the flashing light which told Ms. Escalade to stop, roll down her window, and receive instructions. At 730 a.m., well-ahead of schedule, it was Show Time.

Ms. Escalade and I had been directed into Lane One, which was further good news, because it exactly corresponded to the number **1** on the post-it note on my dashboard. I noticed that none of the cars in front of or behind me had been ushered into Lane 2, and I quickly learned why. Lane 2 was the short line and was populated by the cars that had driven into the facility from the parking lot on the other side of Forest Preserve Drive. Those cars moved through the testing facility at the same slow rate as the cars in front of me. Before I could observe any more Lane 2 activity the Escalade advanced into the first section of the carport's interior and I was waved up to a line of demarcation where a light flashed red.

A woman in Army camouflage, wearing goggles, a face mask, and a face shield knocked on my window. She asked me if the information on my driver's license was correct and if I had written my phone number correctly. I answered yes to both and watched another person peer through the front windshield to copy on his clipboard the information from my i.d. I was given a tissue but not asked to blow my nose. After I repeated my date of birth she said "Okay" and motioned for me to roll down my window and proceed to the next stage of the process.

The Escalade had moved to the center of the building and I was waved further onward, to perhaps three feet from the entrance. With the body of the Escalade out of the way, I had a chance to observe the covey of blue-gowned health care workers gathered just inside the entrance. To my right was the office space annex for the facility. I could see a platoon of U.S. Army personnel in that annex, all in camo, watching the proceedings, moving boxes of supplies to the frontline workers, and disposing of boxes of used supplies from Lane 1.

I guessed that the same coordinated effort was occurring on the far side of Lane 2, but I could not determine how many soldiers, doctors, and nurses were working on that side of the building. If the two lanes operated symmetrically, then the total number of people staffing the site would have exceeded one hundred. It was humbling to think that many people risked their lives each day to administer these tests. I was glad the Army was present to conduct such an orderly, efficient, and trouble-free operation.

When my car was waved inside the building and I saw the dozens of workers in full personal protection equipment, I was reminded of a similar scene in so many science-fiction films I had watched over the decades. Actors in films from <u>Outbreak</u> to <u>Arrival</u> had been similarly garbed when encountering a possible biological threat.

The one film that stood out in my mind as I was directed to advance was Robert Wise's 1971 film <u>The Andromeda Strain</u>. I remembered in <u>The Andromeda Strain</u> that two of the heroes, Dr. Jeremy Stone (Arthur Hill) and Dr. Mark Hall (James Olson) had been dressed in similar hazmat suits when they investigated the source of contamination that had killed nearly all the resident of Piedmont, Arizona. I knew how survivor Peter Jackson (George Mitchell) felt when he spotted the formidably attired Dr. Hall approaching him with a satchel in hand. Mr. Jackson was terrified by what had happened in his hometown and by what Doctor Hall might have in store for him. I shared both fears. What the Coronavirus had done to us was real and problematic; and the sight of these people approaching me without me knowing the exact nature of what I was about to experience was worrisome. Like the one infant that Dr. Stone found alive in Piedmont, I did not know why I was still alive, I could not articulate what was happening to my body, nor did I understand what lay in store for me.

While the medical personnel finished Ms. Escalade's test, the first group of workers wearing baby-blue PPE stood at a tall desk, checking paperwork. One person looked at my driver's license through the windshield and communicating indistinctly with a second group of workers who had now left the Escalade. I was told to advance to where they stood, and upon doing so I was told to turn off the engine and roll down the window. I was not eager to learn if "mildly uncomfortable" was an accurate descriptor, but after all, this early morning exercise had not been arranged for my comfort and convenience. How bad could it be, I wondered. Thousands of people had taken this test and to my knowledge no one had died from it. It could not be as bad as a spinal tap or a prostate ultrasound. I admit those were extreme comparatives, but still, anything less painful than those procedures was okay with me.

I was prepared to be conversational. I always take time to ask how a person's day has been going. I was the only person I could see who was not wearing a face covering, so I smiled at the woman closest to me and said "Good morning, how are you doing? That gown looks great on you. It matches the color of your eyes." I was about to ask her if she was free for lunch or for a drink when her shift ended, but she was all about business and told me "Relax, this will be uncomfortable, but it will be over quick." She said I should "Put your head back against the headrest and hold still."

"So much for foreplay," I thought. I noticed that the conditional "may be uncomfortable" had given way to a definitive and less random "will be uncomfortable." On the other hand, the instruction sheet said it would last for a minute. In my opinion a minute is a relatively long time for such a test, but she had said "quick," and that word was reassuring. I would have preferred her to have said "quickly" but I had learned through experience that it is unwise to correct the grammar of a doctor or nurse who was about to insert something into my body.

As I looked through her face shield and goggles and gazed longingly into her beguiling eyes that were clear as a bright blue sky, I saw a cotton swab coming my way, at the end of a six-inch long stick. I closed my eyes and felt her insert it quickly and gently up the interior of my left sinus passage, further than I had imagined possible. Brad Pitt described the process as a "brain tickling," and his statement was accurate and appropriate. The insertion stimulated a sneeze reflex which was difficult to quash, but I knew that sneezing at such a critical juncture would be unwise and could lead to unfortunate complications. A cerebral hemorrhage was well within the realm of possibilities.

The woman with the swab was true to her word; the collection of a sample was over as quickly as it had begun. I waved goodbye to her and her colleagues and rolled up my window. The last step of the process was to "move to the final station once the test is complete." I assumed that the test was complete because three brave souls were intently occupied with observing, packing, and storing the sample which Ms. Blue Eyes had taken. A fourth person was responsible for spraying and wiping down the area, cleansing it from God knows what might have remained on the tall desk where the others had been working.

What courage it took, I realized, to stand toe to toe with what President Trump was now calling The Hidden Enemy. If I had been a frontline worker, I would have required more stringent measures of protection, on par with the robotic arms Dr. Stone used to manipulate the strain from Andromeda while he was safely ensconced in a cubicle paneled with six inch thick, bulletproof glass. My entire theater of operation would be situated in a sealed, soundproof room like the one in which Raymond Reddington was held captive in the first season of The Blacklist.

Had I been a worker at the Forest Preserve Community-Based Testing Site, at the end of my shift I would have required a decontamination process akin to the one that James Bond and Honey Ryder received after their encounter with the dragon in Dr. No. A naked Ryder and 007 were ushered on a conveyor belt from one scrub-down station to the next of ten such stations. After the tenth stop, they were given a shower and shampoo, followed by an offering of plush terrycloth robes. A final once-over with a Geiger counter made sure every nasty particle of radiation had been removed from their spanking-clean bodies.

I would have requested that a similar process to be in place at no cost to myself before I agreed to work at the Community-Based site. If Dr. No had that technology available to him in 1962, surely fifty-eight years later, the Army would have developed even greater capabilities. I was confident such processes were utilized at all those BSL-4 facilities scattered across our country. If those scientists got the white glove treatment, then certainly the soldiers and health care professionals at Forest Preserve Drive who worked "with agents that could easily be aerosol-transmitted," which could "cause severe to fatal disease in humans for which there are no available vaccines or treatments" deserved the same high level of protection.

I might have waited longer for the "information to take with you" that my leaflet had indicated I would receive before I exited or departed, but when I looked at the second leaflet I recognized what any lamebrain would have quickly deduced. The "information to take with me" was already my hand. By giving me two handouts for the price of one, the Army had acted more efficiently than the leaflet had indicated. An Army sergeant standing near the exit aisle waving me at me, smiling while telling me to get the hell out of his facility, which was ample reassurance that I was done for the day.

I could not believe it was over. My disbelief gave way to palpable elation as I turned left onto Forest Preserve, toward Harlem Avenue and home. To celebrate I took out one of the cds I had brought and went to track four of Buddy Guy's Damn Right I've Got the Blues. The big, quick drum intro and lurid riff of "Mustang Sally" was exactly what I need to clear out the cobwebs. There was no need to wait for the Evening News to see what footage the <u>WGN-TV</u> truck had captured of the events that morning. To discover the status of the people in line who had not arrived by 4 a.m. I made a left turn on Harlem and another on Irving Park. To my and to their eventual dismay, I saw that even if the number of tests to be administered on March 31 had been twice as large as the number of tests performed on March 30, the supply would have been inadequate to service the number of drivers of cars in the queue.

Although I was not hungry, I thought that since I was out in the real world, I should get something to eat for later in the day. I stopped at the Chick-fil-A in Norridge. I figured at 752 a.m. I might have to settle for a chicken breakfast biscuit, but the voice at the drive-through station told me the full menu was available. I ordered the traditional CFA sandwich, which I asked to be prepared plain and without the breading that is typically fried onto their chicken breasts. I had previously researched the topic and had found it did not contain garlic *if* the breading which coated the chicken was eliminated from the formula.

There was no one else in line, which was a pleasant surprise. After I paid my four dollars and fifty-nine cent bill I was told that although breakfast menu items were immediately on hand, I would have to wait ten minutes for a sandwich served more properly at any time of the day other than breakfast time. My requirement of a sandwich sans breading was problematic, but it could be arranged if I waited longer. "Copacetic," I thought. Ten or twenty minutes was a walk in the park compared to how long I had waited on Forest Preserve Drive that morning. To pass the time more pleasantly, I listened to "Hesitation Blues" on my Hot Tuna cd.

Before that acoustic song ended and "How Long Blues" started I realized that, in my haste to get something to eat for later in the day, I had momentarily forgotten how urgently I needed to get home to visit my bathroom. When my sandwich was ready, I thanked the server, grabbed the bag, and found myself pulling into my parking spot before Jorma finished singing his great, live, electric version of "Keep Your Lamp Trimmed and Burning." I did not play the songs as loudly as I would have liked. High numbers of decibels worsened my headaches, but even with the volume tamped down, nothing better soothes an aching body and troubled soul than Kaukonen and Casady blues.

I had observed the speed limit all the way home and I had been careful to watch for other cars, pedestrians, and bicyclists who may not be following the Rules of the Road. A decade ago, I had been struck by a passenger car while I was walking across the street at a four-way-stop intersection. A driver did not heed the red sign and she sent me sprawling into the middle of the intersection. I spent the next few days in the hospital, and I was walking better after six months of physical therapy.

I am mentioning that unfortunate event now because COVID-19 wreaks havoc with one's ability to concentrate. It causes a loss of focus. It is difficult to process time, sequences of events, and memories in an efficient way. Lack of an ability to concentrate is not a good thing to experience when driving. It is far too easy to find your mind drifting without your knowing it. If that happens when driving, the consequences of that inadvertent mental wandering are deadly. I never want to strike a pedestrian, and from March 20-30, I did not drive anywhere. I sincerely urge anyone to refrain from driving while under the influence of the Coronavirus.

I had noticed I was experiencing a corresponding loss of physical balance. I found that standing up without falling over and walking without bumping into things represented ample challenges. It was particularly bitter pill to swallow because for many years before CIDP I had practiced hot yoga, and I had grown proud of my ability to assume one-legged poses without teetering.

I breathed a sigh of relief when I was back in bed that morning. Before relaxing I stowed the chicken sandwich in my refrigerator and drank some ginseng iced green tea. The test was over, thank goodness. I was happy with that accomplishment, but otherwise, I felt terrible. My head was pounding, I was frequently sneezing, my temperature was one hundred and one, and I had constant urge to cough. On top of that I was crashing from a prolonged adrenalin rush.

I found the seesawing nature of my symptoms to be profoundly disturbing. For a few hours each day, perhaps as long as half a day every day for the for the past two weeks, I would feel better and thought my condition had improved, but after each respite the roller coaster of symptoms would return to take me on another ride. The rapid movement from feeling good to experiencing screaming-banshee headaches and feverish heebee-geebee convulsions made COVID-19 more difficult for me to conceptualize and understand. After two weeks of non-static symptoms, I was no longer sure if I was correctly assessing my condition. All I knew was that I was not experiencing a typical flu progression. A dry cough had not migrated into a wet cough; my fever required constant aspirin dosing; and there was no predicting if my next headache would remain a mild distractor or would intensify to attain the magnitude of a blinding migraine.

Since I did not understand the progress of the disease, I did not know what steps to take to treat it. I looked at Sonia, who was sleeping soundly at the foot of my bed. She would have preferred to locate herself nearer to my shoulder, but my fidgeting and restlessness interfered with the sleep pattern which defined two thirds of her day. Her Feline Infectious Peritonitis had been inherited, and its actual cause was a form of the Coronavirus. The disease led to respiratory failure in most cats, usually within a few years of life.

Sonia was seven years old, and I attributed her longevity to the therapies I had employed. I treated her disease as though she were a young child with breathing difficulty. Every morning and evening I gave her a fingertip of a maple-flavored L-Lysine supplement called Viralys. At about 3 p.m. each day I gave her one milliliter of a children's formula decongestant, using any brand that did not contain the active ingredient guaifenesin, which is bad for cats. She liked the Viralys well enough, the decongestant not so much. I administered the decongestant with a plastic syringe commonly used to feed baby birds. I shot the liquid quickly into the back of her throat. It always seemed to work, resulting in her immediately expelling between a half-ounce and an ounce of water and phlegm from her lungs. Her appetite was unimpaired by the procedures and her litterbox activity remained unchanged. An hour after taking the decongestant she was back to her normal, waking activities—watching birds outside the window, attacking the end of my phone-charging cord, and trying to sit on my laptop while I typed.

As I listened to her gentle snoring it dawned on me that there was a lesson to be learned here. Just like Sonia not knowing what FIP was, I did not the first clue about COVID-19's mechanisms of destruction. I wondered what would happen if I treated COVID-19 as though it were a disease with which I was familiar, which was my Chronic Inflammatory Demyelinating

Polyneuropathy. No doctor would prescribe Immunoglobulin infusions to treat COVID-19, but while I had been receiving those infusions, I had developed a supplemental regimen of vitamins and minerals to assist with my recovery. I drank a vegetable smoothie each day, hoping it would help impede the progression of my polyneuropathy.

I could not objectively and independently determine if it was a good or bad idea to attack COVID-19 symptoms this way, but at a gut level I believed that if I could help my immune system battle the disease, it would be worth a try. My alternative was to do nothing, cross my fingers, and hope I did not die, and if I did succumb, to hope I would not die ignominiously, the way those people who were granted an extended stay courtesy of a ventilator had passed.

I enacted the usual safeguards that I would take when coping with the flu. I was drinking fluids, staying warm, and I ate something healthy each night whether I was hungry or not. I took my temperature and blood pressure three times a day. I changed my pajamas, sheets, and pillowcases every other day, and sprayed them each morning with a disinfectant. I used a fresh towel every day. I was careful to keep my hands clean and to dispose of tissues properly so that I would keep from re-infecting myself.

Before doing anything else, I read the second leaflet I had received that morning. These instructions were aimed at **"Tested Healthcare Facility Workers & First Responders,"** but I figured what is good for the goose is good for the gander. The first notation in white print, in an orange box near the top of the page, assured me that **"You will receive a phone call from 1-8338447-0001 with test results in 3-5 days."** Another orange box in the middle of the page clarified that **"When you receive a call for 1-833-447-0001 (Caller ID: Results Center), please answer. Due to privacy considerations, we are unable to leave a message. We will attempt two follow up calls. If you have not received your test result in 7 days, contact your state or local health department."**

That statement seemed curious to me, because the instruction box at top of the page said "**3-5 days**", but the middle-of-the-page instruction box specified "**7 days.**" I glanced at the bottom of that page to make sure it did not say "contact would occur in ten to fourteen days or whenever the hell we get to your case." I was not impressed by the suggestion that if all else fails, **"contact your state or local health department."** My previous attempt to contact IDPH had not been successful, and I had no reason to believe that the process of contacting that department would be easier in any near future attempt. Maybe I would be pleasantly surprised and would receive a phone call in three to five days; maybe I would be told that the test result was negative. Anything was possible, but I viewed both outcomes as equally unlikely.

The other side of that page addressed what would happen next if I tested positive or negative. I thought it prudent to wait a while before memorizing what steps would be appropriate based on test results that I had not yet received.

The rest of the first side of the leaflet addressed four topics. The first was **"What should you do about work while you wait for test results?"** It was a reasonable question, even though it was not relevant to my situation since I worked from home. People who did not work from home were told:

- Please inform your supervisor at work that you have been tested for COVID-19 and note the date of testing.

- If you <u>are experiencing symptoms</u>: Notify your supervisor and stay home.

- If you <u>are not experiencing symptoms</u>: Request guidance from your supervisor on any potential work and patient care restrictions until you know your test results.

- Avoid using public transportation, ride-sharing or taxis when commuting.

I considered this to be straightforward and sage advice. The third bullet point was irrelevant to public at large. It also seemed to me that, unless testing was a job requirement for first responders or health care workers, anyone not experiencing any symptoms of COVID-19 should not have been in line for a test that day. Individuals like myself who were sixty-five years old or greater were required to show symptoms of COVID-19 to qualify for a place in line that day.

The logistics suggested in the fourth bullet point were problematic, because it limited the means of commuting to work to either walking or driving. Driving was a good way to get to work if one is asymptomatic; driving was not a wise choice for anyone who was symptomatic. The instructions did not offer advice about using Uber or Lyft. Perhaps the U.S. Health Service, established in 1798, grouped those two services under the general category of taxis. Many people would read that subpoint could rightfully conclude, "Wow, that's good news, Uber and Lyft are still cool."

Six points were raised under the category of "**What should you do to protect yourself while you wait for test results?**" The first five were accurate and important recommendations:

- Wash your hands often with soap and water for at least 20 seconds. Clean your hands with an alcohol-based hand sanitizer that contains at least 60% alcohol if soap and water are not available.

- Avoid close contact with people who are sick.

- Avoid touching your eyes, nose, and mouth with unwashed hands.

- Clean all "high-touch" surfaces every day. High touch surfaces include counters, tabletops, doorknobs, bathroom fixtures, toilets, phones, keyboards, tablets, and bedside tables.

- Cover coughs and sneezes.

The stipulation of "at least 60% alcohol" was relevant because firms such as Ecolab used 70% ethyl alcohol in their sanitizers, which were made in the USA. Other products of international origin, like the sanitizers made in China, did not meet the sixty percent benchmark, even though those same off-brands claimed ninety-nine-point nine percent effectiveness. The second and fifth points were fine *if* you could differentiate between who was sick and who was not sick. I would be more mindful of the warning in points three and four.

The sixth point was regrettably weak and minimalist in its two qualifications:

- If available, wear a facemask if you are sick.

The only excuse for offering this sixth recommendation is that the U.S. Public Health Service did not know better at the time. Anyone who had listened to President Trump speaking at press conference or at a political rally in Tulsa knew that ignorance is no excuse for disseminating wrong-headed information. If Mr. Trump had not been President I would have expected more from our government. We know that facemasks and coverings used by the public have nothing to do with "**What should you do to protect yourself while you wait for test results.**" Masks and bandanas are employed to help protect others from the disease you might be carrying, not the other way around. The qualifier "If available" would soon become obsolete; that last point should have read "Wear a facemask if you are sick so that you avoid infecting every friend, relative, or total stranger that you may encounter." I wish the woman responsible for The Sneeze would have taken that precaution to heart and would have covered her sneeze, or better still, had stayed home and not used public transportation on that rueful day.

In a light blue box in the lower left corner of the page, five points provided instructions on how to "**Monitor any symptoms.**" These cogent and helpful hints were offered:

- Note the day any new symptoms begin.

- Check your own temperature two times a day.

- Keep a daily record of fever, cough, and additional respiratory symptoms.

- Seek further evaluation from a healthcare provider via telemedicine or an in-person if your symptoms get worse. Call ahead before visiting your doctor and tell them you have been tested for COVID-19.

- Even if you don't experience symptoms, you <u>might</u> make others sick.

At first glance, the third bullet point seemed simple and straightforward, but it contained a stereotypically reductive fallacy. Keeping an accurate taxonomy of symptoms is a complex and difficult task to achieve when in the throes of COVID-19. Four main factors increase the level of difficulty. First, it is hard to assess the severity of old symptoms and the presence of new ones because the symptoms change so frequently. Second, COVID-19 throws askew one's normal mental agility, making it a challenge to recognize and remember to record various symptoms of the disease. Third, Coronavirus symptoms come in waves. They are not discrete events that can be metrically recorded. Finally, it is difficult to maintain the motivation necessary to keep these types of lists. It is emotionally draining to fight off constant chills, fevers, coughs, headaches, and congestion. When I could not breathe in the middle of some nights, the last thing I wanted to do was turn on a light, take out my notebook, and scribble in a way that may not be legible in the morning that at 246 a.m. I felt like I was going to die because I could not catch my breath. There were many occasions when I was betrayed by the faulty belief that I would remember what happened in the morning.

I developed a work-around which I admit was not perfect, but it was one that allowed me to maintain an accurate record of symptoms for posterity. I assigned a number value ranging from one to five, with one corresponding to a very mild fever, an intermittent cough, or an uncomfortable but not disabling additional respiratory symptom like an inability to clear my throat or a slight gagging when I tried to breathe deeply. A five rating would mean that, if a symptom's severity continued for more than a minute, I should call 911.

I revised my numbers as the days passed based on how I felt. For example, if I originally thought a cough rated a four and later found out what a four really meant, I would cross of the four and make it a two or three. The quantification of symptoms allowed me to graph the results, and I could watch with some dismay as my graph resembled the first half of bell-shaped curve. I found that keeping the log and adding points to the graphs did not make me feel better, but it temporarily distracted me from the unpleasantness of the symptoms I was faithfully charting.

The advice in the bullet point about seeking a "further evaluation via telemedicine" sounded like I should consult some version of WebMD to receive an evaluation, but I can assure you, no such facility exists for COVID-19. I could not find a dedicated website; I could not participate in a Zoom workshop where a doctor would tell me, for example, "Well, you've had that cough for three days, so here's how you should think about that." I would have preferred if that bullet point had read "via telemedicine or via an in-person appointment with Doctor Who when you will be told to Stay Calm and proceed to your nearest Tardis."

The implication of the phrase "before visiting your doctor and tell them" irritated me. Did the U.S. Public Health Service believe that, like President Trump, I had a team of doctors at my beck and call? My doctor was a singular person, not a collective "them." Why hadn't they hired a proofreader for God's sake? But these minor idiomatic transgressions were redeemed by the posit, "you <u>might</u> make others sick." Perhaps the writer or editor had gone too far by underlining "might." It was a judgement call I was not be prepared to make until three, five, or seven days later.

While it is true that those last two points under the topic "**Monitor any symptoms**" extended far and beyond the general category of "monitoring symptoms," a navy-blue box to its immediate right contained instructions which upped the ante. It listed the extremes of symptoms that I would rate as fours or fives. That box of instructions in the lower right-hand corner of the page told me to "**Seek medical attention immediately if you develop any sign of the following emergency warning signs for COVID-19 or other medical emergencies**." Those emergency signs consisted of:

- Extremely difficult breathing

- Bluish lips or face

- Constant pain or pressure in the chest

- Severe constant dizziness or lightheadedness

- Acting confused

- Difficult to wake up

- Slurred speed (new or worsening)

- New seizure or seizures that won't stop

These items did not seem to me to be "warning signs." Their gravity extended far beyond "**warning signs for COVID-19.**" These were indices that there was no longer any need to worry about a possible COVID-19 infection because Last Rites should be administered as quickly as possible. According to that list, though, by my count I should have called 911 four times, having qualified on points one, four, five, and six.

Regarding point five, "**Acting confused,**" I should point out that I was not *acting*, I was experiencing the genuine article. I was not **Acting confused** if I forgot to turn off one of the electric burners on my stovetop. The consequences for my genuine absentmindedness would have been one hundred percent real. I hoped that the other two hundred and fifty people who received this brochure on March 31 held themselves to a higher degree of accountability and did not call 911 when they noticed they had changed lanes while driving without looking to see if another car occupied the same space they would soon be entering, or when they walked into their kitchens twice before remembering why they entered the kitchen the first time, or when they found themselves having to rewind the dvr for the fifth time because they could not recall what had transpired in the two minute opening scene of <u>Chicago Med</u>.

The sixth crucial indicator, **Difficult to wake up**, addressed an event I encountered several times each day. I deduced that the person who wrote this brochure did not have a personal encounter with COVID-19. In that regard the person was extremely fortunate.

Regarding the warning sign of **Slurred speed (new or worsening)**, since I could not talk without coughing, I stopped talking to myself, and consequently my speech was not slurred. I was not aware of making any verbal gaffs when I spoke to Sonia, but it is easy to vocalize "Hi Sonia!" or "Here kitty kitty!" without mispronouncing those words. I had no trouble enunciating the words in the simple questions I put to her, such as, "What would you prefer for dinner, my dear? Perhaps some yummy Fancy Feast Creamy Delights Chicken Feast with a touch of Real Milk In A Creamy Sauce? Or would a fresh can of Fancy Feast Gourmet Naturals White Meat Chicken Recipe be more to your liking?" Those words were so often repeated by me that I could say them in my sleep without slurring.

The unsettling disclaimers "**This list is not all-inclusive**" and "**Please consult your medical professional for any other symptoms that are severe or concerning**" ran underneath the listing of those eight extreme symptoms. I could not imagine how I could survive symptoms on a more inclusive list, or how the symptoms listed could be more severe. The concept that those two possibilities existed was scarier to me than the notion of being forced to stand on the cantilevered, glass-floored Ledge on the one hundred and third floor of the Willis Tower and look down.

The first of two lines at the bottom of the page repeated the protocol to follow in case of a medical emergency. The instruction had been repeated so often that Sonia probably knew when to call 911. The second line provided a bit of new information, stating "**FOR MORE INFORMATION VISIT: <u>WWW.CORONAVIRUS.GOV</u>**." Anyone who visits that site will not learn new and exciting information about the Coronavirus. I found nothing there that lessened my level of anxiety or increased my store of knowledge. The website is in fact the source work for the suggestions and instructions that I found on the two leaflets I received at the Community-Based Testing Site. It was fun to look at the smiling faces in the colorful pictures found on the website, but because I was hoping to find something more profound and meaningful, perhaps answers to the questions like "how high of a fever should I have to warrant a 911 call" or "what is causing me to cough so frequently," I left the site more depressed than I was before visiting it.

Before planning what incremental measures I could take to mitigate or end the presence of the Coronavirus in my body, I thought it prudent to figure out and list the things I *absolutely should not* do. A plentiful supply of misinformation existed about Coronavirus and how to cure COVID-19, and I needed to look at all of it, because I could not afford to miss out on a promising therapy. I would search the house where the Coronavirus dwelled "room by room, patiently," as Audioslave described in its song "Like a Stone." I needed to explore every nook and cranny of its dark real estate. I would discover that most of those rooms would be empty. Though they might lack any sensible offering, misinformation could be useful because, as in any maze, dead ends force backtracking, which could suggest a more successful avenue of approach.

I was not yet delusional enough to surmise that I could find a solution to a pandemic that has stumped the greatest scientific minds of our century. My only goal was to stay alive, to find a way to avoid the death that had already taken tens of thousands of American lives. I was desperate to avoid a COVID-19-only intensive care unit, which I irrationally viewed as our contemporary equivalent of a Solzhenitsyn ward. It would be a big win if I could minimize my symptoms enough to obviate a need for intubations and ventilators.

Proposed cures for COVID-19 ranged from the sublime to the ridiculous, heavily weighted toward the latter. A promising, elegant solution, according to Dr. Fauci, might be the drug Rmdesivir. At the Task Force briefing of February 7 he stated, "What they're looking at is the effect of this drug — either the drug plus standard of care versus standard of care alone." He also described the process for developing vaccines for the Coronavirus. He explained, "One of the first steps is to successfully get that (novel coronavirus) gene and insert it into the messenger RNA platform successfully and allow it to express proteins. We've succeeded in that. The next (step) is to put it in a mouse animal model to induce immunogenicity, and to get the company to make (gold nanoparticle) products. All of those have been successfully implemented. There have been no glitches so far. If that continues, we will be in Phase 1 trials in people within the next two-and-a-half months."[1] If we could afford to show "a little patience," as Axl Rose had once sung, our scientific community might solve the problem sooner than me might otherwise expect.

In Okeechobee County, Florida, an impatient County Board Commissioner Bryant Culpepper was not a Guns 'n' Roses fan. He had noticed that test samples were gathered using nasal swabs. He asserted that if someone—not himself, by the way—applied heat to nasal passages, "the coolest part of the body" where the Coronavirus settled before migrating to the lungs, that emboldened person could quickly kill the virus. Following his Wile E. Coyote logic to its natural conclusion, Culpepper recommended heating those sinus passages by holding a hair dryer against one's face, and turning it on so that it could heat one's nostrils to an optimal one hundred and thirty-three degrees.

When called on the carpet to defend such an inspired protocol, he first falsely asserted that he had quoted a report he had seen on One America

News. When that news network denied his allegation, and after the World Health Organization warned the only results one could reliably expect from such a procedure were charred nasal membranes and burnt corneas, Culpepper stood his ground. Aware of his responsibility as a civil servant and mindful of upcoming elections, he later added "I was only trying to give comfort to those in Okeechobee who have no insurance to treat there (sic) families."[2] Tempting as it sounded, I was able to resist that remedy because I did not own a hair dryer.

The government official voted Least Likely to Join the Guns 'n' Roses Fan Club was our Treasury Secretary Steve Mnuchin. Proving that he was every bit the curmudgeon we suspected him to be, Steve kicked off the biggest government vs. rocker feud since the 1985 Senate Commerce, Science, and Transportation Committee Hearings, when Dee Snider of Twisted Sister and Frank Zappa battled Tipper Gore and Susan Baker's Parents Resource Music Center on the topic of censorship of rock music.

The PRMC had developed a list of "Filthy Fifteen" rock songs. Senator Slade Gorton told Zappa, "You could manage to give the First Amendment to the Constitution of the United States a bad name if I felt you had the slightest understanding of it, which I do not." Senator Paula Hawkins chided Van Halen for obscenity in its songs. To prove her point, she required senators to watch the group's 1984 music video "Hot for Teacher." She did not define why "Hot for Teacher" was more suggestive than many Chuck Berry songs she and her teenage friends had listened to at the local Happy Days malt shop when they were young. Such an explanation would have forced Paula and Tipper and Susan to admit to the popular music-loving world that they were hypocrites.

Axl Rose's previous encounter with our government's mishandling of a crisis occurred in 2018, when he took issue with President Trump's blaming the California's Department of Forestry for the destruction caused by wildfires. Rose tweeted, "Um...actually...it's a lack of federal funding that's at the 'root' of the purported forest mismanagement. Only a demented n' truly pathetic individual would twist that around 'n' use a tragedy to once again misrepresent facts for attempted public/political gain at other's expense."

On May 5, when President Trump toured the Phoenix, Arizona Honeywell factory, one of the songs playing over the factory's public address system was Guns 'n' Roses version of "Live and Let Die." Factory officials were aware that when Mr. Trump campaigned for the Presidency, he would sometimes play Guns 'n' Roses songs at rallies. The Honeywell managers believed choosing "Live and Let Day" would be an appropriate and welcome gesture, a nod to his successful tenure in office.

This choice of a soundtrack was to say the least ironic, scripted better than anyone except Axl Rose himself could have managed. Though he could not prevent Honeywell or President Trump from using his songs as they saw fit, he was no friend of the current Administration. He made his own political opinion clear when, *prior to* the Coronavirus pandemic, he tweeted "Trump administration along w/the majority of Republicans in Congress n' their donors that support him 4 their own agendas r doing r nation a disservice. We have an individual in the WH that will say n' do anything w/no regard for truth, ethics, morals or empathy of any kind, who says what's real is fake n' what's fake is real, who will stop at nothing 4 power feeding off the anger n' resentment he sows 24/7 while constantly whining how whatever doesn't go his way is unfair...Most of us in America have never experienced anything this obscene at this level in r lifetimes n' if we as a country *don't wake up* n' put an end 2 this nonsense now *it's something we definitely will all pay hard 4 as time goes on.*"

The Honeywell plant had been retrofitted to produce masks. Signs were posted throughout the facility requiring everyone to wear a mask. The President refused to comply. Despite considerable blowback resulting from his defiance of that company's policy, no lesson was learned. On May 21 he toured a Ford plant in Ypsilanti, Michigan, and refused to wear a mask, even though the facility was making masks, not cars.

Two days later, thousands of social-distancing protestors kicked off Memorial Day weekend by not wearing masks when they gathered on hundreds of Illinois street corners in large groups, in defiance of state laws prohibiting such gatherings. The protestors held patently banal signs while shouting trumped-up clichés at passing cars. Some of the signs read "Freedom Not Flu." I was not aware that such a binary existed, nor could I determine any hidden meaning in the sentiment. Other signs read "Pritzker Sucks" and "Transition to Greatness." To underscore a blatantly obvious political point, none of the protestors wore masks. Such was the deadly effect of leadership by example.

I assumed that none of the protestors were students of history. Like President Trump, they had no awareness that during the Spanish Flu, the governor of Missouri ordered that the city of St. Louis be completely shut down, while the city of Philadelphia welcomed all brethren with open arms, hosting parades, fairs, and picnics in the parks. A few months later, St. Louis had one of the lowest rates of death from Spanish Flu of all U.S. major cities, while Philadelphia posted one of the highest rates.

Social-distancing protestors also seemed capable of ignoring current affairs. For example, large groups of Texans, hellbent on whooping it up on Memorial Day weekend, gathered at square-dances, at rodeos, and on spring break beaches they had visited a month earlier. By the end of May, the number of positive Coronavirus tests in Houston skyrocketed from two hundred a day to two thousand per day.

The attitude of vacationers on South Padre Island that weekend made this leap of faith understandable. A twenty-something sand and surf celebrant expressed his gleeful confidence that the Coronavirus was not real—he thought the pandemic was a practical joke perpetrated by deluded scientists who meant to stop him from having a Good Time. He asked why the reporter was wearing a face covering. When he was told "To protect myself and you," the young man replied, "You don't need a mask to do that; all you have to do is not touch your face." The man who did not appear to be as intoxicated as his nearby friends began touching his mouth, nose, eyes, and cheeks. No matter how many other people wore face coverings, a mask would not be part of his beach attire. His televised interview provided a good example of "Freedom not Flu" irrationality.

A similar attitude was expressed by our Secretary of Treasury. The Center for Disease Control warned us that "Travel increases your chances of getting and spreading COVID-19—CDC recommends you stay home as much as possible, especially if your trip is not essential, to avoid higher risk of severe illness." Steve Mnuchin expressed a contrary opinion when on May 4 he stated, "This is a great time for people to explore America. A lot of people haven't seen many parts of America. The President's also looking about ways to stimulate travel. We want people to travel safely, to be able to visit places safely." Upon hearing Mnuchin's statement, one which Axl Rose figured was counterintuitive to the notion of protecting the American public, the singer tweeted on May 6, "It's official! Whatever anyone may have previously thought of Steve Mnuchin, he's officially an asshole."

Mnuchin felt empowered to reply to Rose's tweet by asking the singer "What have you done for this country lately?" To gild that lily Steve added a flag icon. Unfortunately, our Cabinet member had included a picture of the flag of Liberia in this tweet, not an American flag. Axl noticed the inappropriateness of both the question Mnuchin posed and the flag he had included, and replied, "My bad I didn't get we're hoping 2 emulate Liberia's economic model but on the real unlike this admin I'm not responsible for 70k+ deaths n' unlike u I don't hold a fed gov position of responsibility 2 the American people n' go on TV tellin them 2 travel the US during a pandemic." The reply left Mnuchin befuddled. He was too stupid to rue the day he left Hollywood to accept the job as the official White House asshole, a position for which there was a surfeit of competition.

Meanwhile, a possible remedy had surfaced, one which I favored but sadly one in which I could not partake. A bold experimenter reported that drinking garlic water and eating garlic would cure COVID-19. Spurred on by this news, a woman from China ate three point three pounds of garlic. No one had told her that "A 1.0 g/kg body weight/day dose of garlic was associated with marked histological damage in liver."[3] Needless to say, China attributed her death to ancillary liver damage, not to the Coronavirus she had hoped to kill by eating one and a half kilos of garlic.

When it was falsely reported that Five-G antennae were spreading the Coronavirus, sleepy London Town's street fighting men took to neighboring fields on search and destroy missions. The New York Times reported that "On April 2, a wireless tower was set ablaze in Birmingham. The next day, a fire was reported at 10 p.m. at a telecommunications box in Liverpool. An hour later, an emergency call came in about another cell tower in Liverpool that was going up in flames. Across Britain, more than 30 acts of arson and vandalism have taken place against wireless towers and other telecom gear this month, according to police reports and a telecom trade group."[4]

Any self-respecting conspiracy theorist knows that a Five-G network causes headaches and brain tumors, not COVID-19. Once again, conspiracy activists got their facts one hundred and eighty degrees wrong. They should have directed their energies toward building more Five G towers to kill the Coronavirus, not wasting their time and effort destroying the precious few still standing. Microwave towers are helpful for stopping, not spreading an alien incursion, as proven in Chris Gorak's 2011 film The Darkest Hour.

There are other many ways that microwaves could be employed to combat this disease. In his cult film Microwave Massacre, if COVID-19 existed in 1979, director Wayne Berwick could have used microwaves to kill the Coronavirus that lived inside a COVID-19 crab sandwich. The character in the lead role, who was coincidentally named Donald, would have found that eating a microwaved crab sandwich was heathier and tastier than snacking on parts of his deceased wife's corpse, which had provided him with a few gruesomely filling meals.

A current and eminently more practical application for microwaves involved the alleged transmission of the Coronavirus by mail. I read that I should microwave my mail before touching or opening any envelopes. I was aware that microwaves use extremely short-lived waves of radiation to cook food items with heat.

I did not think that microwaving my mail was necessary, because I believed that baking my mail at three hundred and fifty degrees for fifty minutes in my conventional oven was a more efficient way to kill any errant Coronavirus nanoparticles. My traditional oven would consistently outperform my microwave oven if I heated my mail because microwaves ovens cook items unevenly. When I thaw and heat my Lou Malnati's pizza in my microwave, for example, some parts are always hotter than others, but when cooked properly in my Classic Series Frigidaire conventional oven, not only is the pizza uniformly hot, it is also crispy, which is a texture impossible to attain when I use my Frigidaire FMV1 Convenient Cooking microwave oven.

If I accepted the far-fetched notion that the Coronavirus is living and breathing in my next Com Ed bill or lurking within the shadows of my next Victoria's Secret catalog—which I receive to keep abreast of current fashion trends and to allow me to speak knowledgeably when the topic of female undergarments arises in discussions with the waitresses at Countryside—the microwaving of that literature would not be one hundred percent effective.

For example, after two minutes of microwaving, some pages in the lipstick ads in the magazine might be at or near room temperature, while other pages in the see-through swimwear section might be too hot to handle. Also, if I did not screen my mail carefully, I would risk burning out my microwave unit and possibly starting a housefire if I heated for more than ten seconds a solicitation that had a nickel enclosed, for me to keep whether or not I donated fifty dollars to the Sierra Club. After I watched Michael Moore's recent film, <u>Planet of the Humans</u>, I knew I would never become a Sierra Club supporter.

When I received my twelve-hundred dollar check from President Trump to compensate me for my loss of work, I did not take a chance of burning it to a crisp in my microwave or charring it in my electric oven. In South Korea, mindful citizens microwaved many paper products to protect themselves from infection. They abruptly halted that process when they realized that "trying to sterilize their cash in the microwave caused it to begin disintegrating."[5]

Because breast milk has been found to protect most infants from measles and chickenpox for a while after birth, some men, probably those with breast fixations, declared that breast milk would protect them from COVID-19. More fuel to that fire was added when the Center for Disease Control and Prevention stated "mother-to-child transmission of Coronavirus during pregnancy is unlikely." Breast milk proponents neglected to consider the CDC's disclaimer "but after birth, a newborn is susceptible to person-to-person spread."[6] If a breast-feeding infant could be infected with the Coronavirus, then breast milk was not protecting the infant from COVID-19. Nor would it protect any other child or adult from the Coronavirus.

Major General Hossein Salami, who was an independent entrepreneur when he was not occupied leading Iran's Islamic Revolutionary Guard Corps, marketed a forty-thousand-dollar COVID-19 detector, invented by fellow countryman and Class-A conman Shayan Sardarizadeh. Salami claimed the Rube Goldberg device "can detect the coronavirus in a few seconds, from a distance of 330 feet" without having to "draw blood or get close enough to the potentially infected patient."[7] He hyped Sardarizadeh's invention as "an amazing scientific technique that has been tested across various hospitals."

After a few weeks of brisk sales to wealthy Iranians and to Middle East government representatives, Salami took a break from his sales liaison position to address the more touch-and-go matter of Iranian gunboats and their interactions with our Fifth Fleet. He stated, "We declare to the Americans that we are absolutely determined and serious...and that all action will be met with a decisive response that will be efficient and quick."[8] Coincidentally, sales of the Salami Slammer sank after those recent gunboat incursions.

France's Health Minister Olivier Veran told his constituents not to take aspirin or ibuprofen because those products "worsened symptoms of the illness caused by the coronavirus."[9] According to Dr. Michele Barry at Stanford's Center for Innovation in Global Health, "There is no reason to think that infected patients should avoid temporary use of ibuprofen."[10]

Our own homespun advocates of nonscientific Coronavirus-killing methodologies would not be upstaged by phony garlic, microwave, breast milk, or aspirin theatrics. For example, if garlic could defeat the virus, certainly its vampire-repellant counterpart, silver, would function equally well in abating the Coronavirus. One such advocate of drinking colloidal silver is Jordan Sather, who tweeted that "Colloidal Silver is more of a sword than a shield, to put it metaphorically. It kills." He was correct. Drinking silver does kill, but the victim is the poor fool who followed his recommendation. Silver is but one of Sather's Miracle Mineral Supplements. MMS's active ingredient is "chlorine dioxide–a bleaching agent."[11]

It's hard to imagine that anyone would take his nonsense seriously, but one of Sather's followers re-tweeted "It's on the list of viruses that MMS can handle. No wonder they are suppressing MMS so hard." By "it" this person meant the Coronavirus, and by "they" we can assume the reference is to Big Pharma, which is an entity Sather believes "wants you ignorant" of his remarkably life-affirming product.

Depending on the size of the dose, silver can cause mild side effects such as argyria, which means one's "skin turns a bluish gray as granules of silver accumulate in the body," or severe one, because "the conjunctiva and internal organs may also be affected." The condition is permanent because "Once silver is deposited, there's no way to get it out."

If the silver dosage is large enough—and who would want to scrimp on a Sather-endorsed product—it can lead to "kidney damage, stomach distress, and headaches," followed by "brain and nerve damage (resulting) from silver exposure."[12] As if these deterrents weren't crazy enough, President Trump endorsed one more vampire-killing element, sunlight, as a potent remedy in this neo-Stoker world of hypothetical Coronavirus combat.

I was surprised to learn that gargling with salt water, vinegar, or lemon juice would defeat the Invisible Enemy. Once more, the Center for Disease Control countered that theory with facts, leading WebMD to explain that the Coronavirus "enters your body when you breathe in virus that's floating in the air after it was coughed or sneezed by an infected person. Another way the virus gains entry into our body is when we touch our nose with our hands contaminated with virus. In both instances, the virus *never lands* in the part of the throat that gargling would even touch."[13]

Though staying hydrated is always a good idea, especially when suffering from rampant COVID-19 fever, drinking a glass of water every fifteen minutes is not an effective weapon in the battle against the Coronavirus. Drinking water cannot kill the Coronavirus, even though it has been claimed that "water and other liquids can flush it away, into your stomach where it cannot survive because of your stomach acid...if you don't drink water often enough, the coronavirus will get into your airways and then into your lungs."[14]

If the Coronavirus had made its way to my throat, I could reasonably assume it had also been present in my nasal passages, and probably had already infiltrated my lungs. Since that was the case, even if I drank gallons of Propel Vitamin Water every fifteen minutes, the liquid would have no effect on the Coronavirus. Since the Coronavirus is transmitted as an aerosol, and not as an after-dinner mint, drinking will not exempt it from getting into my airways and then into my lungs, nor will it force the virus out of my nasal passages and into my stomach. I did not want the

Coronavirus anywhere near my stomach. Anyone who has seen Ridley Scott's Alien can understand my trepidation over sharing John Hurt's fate.

Warm weather will not kill the Coronavirus, contrary to President Trump's stated position that "the (summer) heat generally speaking kills this kind of virus." No friend to his fictions, the World Health Organization reported that "the coronavirus can be transmitted in all areas of the globe, including hot climates. It won't just go away in the Northern Hemisphere as the weather gets warmer in spring and summer."[15]

I remember that in my childhood, on a hot summer day nothing was more refreshing than a Good Humor ice cream bar. Even now when I hear bells jingling, I do not think of Christmas or the Carol of the Bells—my first impulse is to go to my freezer and eat half a container of Ben and Jerry's AmeriCone Dream. In a bit of good news for our beleaguered and dessert-loving President, the tenet that avoiding ice cream will protect us from the Coronavirus was debunked by the humanitarian organization he detested. The W.H.O. stated, "There is no scientific evidence that eating hygienically made frozen food and ice-cream spreads the new coronavirus."[16]

I often held my breath as I waited for that Good Humor truck to roll closer to my parents' home in Edison Park. Contrary to the statements made by Al Capone vault exhumer Geraldo Rivera, my ability to hold my breath is not a reliable replacement for getting a COVID-19 test.[17] Holding his breath was as effective for Geraldo in 2020 as it was in 2016, when he waited with bated breath to be rewarded for his performance with Edyta Sliwinska on ABC's Dancing with the Stars. Rivera and Sliwinska were the first of Season Twenty-Two contestants to be eliminated from the competition.

Homemade sanitizers will not kill the Coronavirus for two reasons: either they will lack the requisite percentage of alcohol, or quality control will not be of laboratory grade. An intrepid New York Times reporter thought she would try the Do It Yourself approach. She was not pleased with the results when she concocted a bowl of goo that failed to pass muster. She described what happened when she donned her lab coat, stating "Mostly I just made a mess. After mixing alcohol and aloe vera gel in a bowl, the mix created weird globules, and the gel began to separate and sink to the bottom. After mixing a few more times, the final product was runny and more like straight alcohol than the easy-to-apply gel I was hoping for. (And after a few hours it began to separate again.)"[18]

It has been suggested that drinking sesame oil, drinking cow urine, taking massages with essential oils, bathing in extremely hot or ice-cold water, inhaling fumes from burning sage, ingesting fifty milligrams of cannabis edibles, taking antibiotics, using steroids, drinking alcohol to excess, avoiding flies and mosquitos, not eating Chinese food, and not touching packages shipped from China are effective preventive and therapeutic measures. None of those claims have any merit. Most of those ludicrously-false assertions receive national attention because "when the word 'pandemic' starts appearing in headlines, people become fearful — and with fear comes misinformation and rumors."[19]

As is always the case, unscrupulous wraiths prey on and profit from fear. For example, I watched a news report about the Tower of Babel that we commonly refer to as Tele-Evangelism. It showed various preachers declaring that they could blow the wind of God into me to kill COVID-19 if I provided them with an appropriate tithe. As a bonus offer, if I made payment to the First Church of the Mountebanks within the next three hours, a second tele-parishioner friend of mine would receive via USPS mail a his or her own Saving Breath, free of charge, if I paid an additional handling fee. Taxes and shipping costs were not included on the bonus offer. I know that our prayers to God are always answered, but any offering I made to these charlatans to cure COVID-19-did not have a prayer of a chance of succeeding.

Realizing that my research had shown me the tip of the iceberg, I asked myself how those people who were responsible for fact-checking all these claims about Coronavirus "remedies" were handling what seemed to be a massive daily influx of misinformation. The obvious answer to my question was "not too well." A fact-check team manager employed by the German firm Correctiv revealed that "It's a really hard job to monitor all of this stuff and stay emotionally stable. When you stop the work in the evenings, you turn on the TV and what do you see? More coronavirus."

After sorting through rumors that the Coronavirus was part of a plot by the United States to use Bosnia as a base to invade Russia, a Balkan fact-checker admitted, "I'm not holding up well. It's hard to decompress." An employee of the Spanish firm Matilda described how her company "is now getting 2,000 daily submissions from people flagging potential misinformation on WhatsApp, up from 250 queries before the pandemic began." In our country, a fact-checker with FirstDraft believed that "Local news is probably, in the name of trying to be helpful, the worst in spreading misinformation."[20]

The increased use of social media to spread misinformation about the Coronavirus exacerbates the problems that fact-checkers encounter. One consultant stated, "While a social medium has many advantages, such as the ability to deliver news instantly, reaching different audiences faster, it also creates huge problems, such as fake news."[21] The problem of global "rampant misinformation" has become so severe that "The World Health Organization now classifies this issue as an infodemic."[22] The International Fact Checking Network of the Poynter Institute, an organization which "unites more than 100 fact-checkers around the world in publishing, sharing and translating facts surrounding the new coronavirus," broke the story of the infodemic. The Network has recently proved the accuracy of a "rumor" that "restaurants have started tacking a COVID-19 surcharge onto customer's bills."[23]

Facebook and other platforms have claimed to be working hard to solve the spread of fictional claims about the Coronavirus, but many experts fear that the sheer bulk of misinformation has caused an unsolvable problem. One expert in biology and in the science of misinformation at the University of Washington, Professor Carl Bergstrom, believes that efforts to stop the spread "are too little, too late." He stated that social media conglomerates have "built this whole ecosystem that is all about engagement, allows viral spread, and hasn't ever put any currency on accuracy. Now all of a sudden we have a serious global crisis, and they want to put some Band-Aids on it. It's better than not acting, but praising them for doing it is like praising Philip Morris for putting filters on cigarettes."[24] The self-policing efforts of social media giants have been attacked by President Trump, who claimed that his tweets , which contain a constant barrage ludicrous assertions, have been unjustly censored.

On March 22, the major media source of misinformation in our country, Fox News, stated that with the federal government had supplied states with ten million Coronavirus tests in the first two weeks of March, and as many as twenty-seven million more tests stood at the ready.[25] This news came on the heels of a March 21 <u>CNN</u> report quoting Dr. Deborah Brix, who said that one hundred and seventy-thousand United States residents had been tested. In that same report Dr. Fauci was asked if the government has met the demand for tests from states, he replied "We are not there yet."[26]

On March 26, Governor Cuomo asked for additional ventilators. Later that night, after Sean Hannity had reported that Governor Cuomo was wrong and New York did not need more ventilators, President Trump told Hannity "I have a feeling that a lot of the numbers that are being said in some areas are just bigger than they're going to be." President Trump declared "I don't believe you need 40,000 or 30,000 ventilators. You go into major hospitals sometimes, and they'll have two ventilators. And now, all of a sudden, they're saying, 'Can we order 30,000 ventilators?'"[27] These are but two illustrations of the curious interaction that has been become known as the "feedback loop between Fox and Trump."[28]

To understand how this "feedback loop" works, imagine President Trump watching a <u>Fox News</u> report about the Coronavirus and then tweeting out those erroneous "facts." Then picture <u>Fox News</u> reporting the tweets, but not mentioning where the President might have received the information he was publicly acknowledging as facts. The <u>Fox News</u> report implied that the President had secret knowledge about the topic. Perhaps this knowledge arose from his Daily President's Briefings, had he bothered to read them. Perhaps he had a secret meeting with Jared Kushner. Any source *except* <u>Fox News</u> could have provided the President with these new "facts."

The feedback loop began when Donald Trump campaigned for the Presidency. Mathew Gertz, a senior fellow at Media Matters for America, has tracked hundreds of examples of the loop phenomenon since then. Thanks to the "'Super TiVo' that was installed at the White House,"[29] President Trump typically reviews hours of "Fox & Friends" each day, resulting in his "hyperaggressive early morning tweetstorms."[30]

The most blatant recent example of this marriage of convenience was the Laura Ingraham/Tucker Carlson hype of the drug hydroxychloroquine. On March 20 Ingraham called the drug a "game-changer" which would provide COVID-19 patients with a "miracle turnaround." On March 21 President Trump tweeted "HYDROXYCHLOROQUINE & AZITHROMYCIN, taken together, have a real chance to be one of the biggest game changers in the history of medicine."[31]

On March 21 Tucker Carlson climbed on the bandwagon, touting the drug and stating "Several days ago, the President expressed confidence in hydroxychloroquine as a treatment for the epidemic. Donald Trump is not the only person who thinks hydroxychloroquine might be effective. A lot of practicing physicians think so, too."[32] The fallacy in Carlson's contorted *argumentum ad hominem* was ignored. No one asked for the names and qualifications of that lot of practicing physicians. On March 24, the Center for Disease Control said that both unauthorized and medically supervised uses of hydroxychloroquine were dangerous. From March 21 onward though, President Trump ignored the recommendations of knowledgeable sources and sided with Tucker Carlson who had no scientific background and who, like Geraldo Rivera, had failed as a contestant on Dancing with the Stars. This unsettlingly career path prepared Carlson to dance flat-footed with Donald Trump.

On April 22, the damning results of a Veteran's Administration trial of hydroxychloroquine were released, which showed that more deaths occurred in a group that took the drug than in a control group. First Fox, then the President retreated from supporting the use of the drug. Two days later, our Janus-faced President Trump tweeted that he would like to "flood" the New York and New Jersey with hydroxychloroquine, a move upon which Ingraham and Carlson waxed favorably.

By then millions of Americans had requested prescriptions for hydroxychloroquine. One couple in their sixties chose not to wait for help from their doctor and their pharmacist. They had a ready supply of hydroxychloroquine phosphate in a cabinet next to their aquarium. Though they were not ill, they decided to use the drug for two reasons: it worked well enough to kill fish parasites, and the President thought it was a promising remedy. The woman later stated, "I saw it sitting on the back shelf and thought, 'Hey, isn't that the stuff they're talking about on TV? We were afraid of getting sick."[33] The couple created a hydroxychloroquine cocktail for themselves, and down their gullets it went.

Things went awry, as they invariably will whenever a chemical substance of unknown quality is ingested using a "best-guess" approach to the size of a dosage. The man died after he arrived at a hospital. The bereaved widow "was initially in critical condition but is now stable and expected to fully recover."[34]

The President expressed no remorse, because he did not acknowledge that the event had anything to do with his enthusiastic outbursts about the use of hydroxychloroquine. On May 18 President Trump offered us a whole-hearted endorsement of hydroxychloroquine. He stunned reporters at a press conference and the rest of the rational world by revealing that he had started taking hydroxychloroquine "a couple weeks ago" as a preventive measure. He said he began swallowing the prophylactic perhaps as early as May 8 when the Vice President's press secretary Katie Miller tested positive for COVID-19. The President's decision to take this drug was based on "a lot of tremendously positive news on the hydroxy." Whether he took the drug, or just claimed he had done so remains an open question. Either way, his statement was geared to encourage more Americans to take hydroxychloroquine. He underlined the safety of his approach by stating unceremoniously, "so far I seem to be OK."

Americans do not have access to a corps of doctors providing us with twenty-four-hour a day medical supervision, which was a detail the President neglected to mention. Even when administered under strict medical supervision, the use of hydroxychloroquine has since proved to be ineffective. Thanks to mutually-beneficial financial deals that link President Trump and Jared Kushner to Sanofi, the French firm that produces hydroxychloroquine, the United States now possesses sixty million doses of the drug, and we are well-prepared to combat a malaria outbreak, the next time it threatens the health and well-being of our citizenry. President Trump was well-motivated to tweet on July 7, "HYDROXYCHLOROQUINE cut the death rate in certain sick patients very significantly. The Dems disparaged it for political reasons (me!). Disgraceful. Act now." The "disgraceful" part of his sentiment applied to his hawking of the dangerous drug, using the same "Act Now!" tactic that Popeil used to sell its Pocket Fisherman, that Suzanne Somers used to sell her Thigh Master, that Vince Shlomi used to sell the Slap Chop.

The President learned nothing from the outrage that arose when he made a similarly irresponsible series of statements a month earlier, ones which shocked the entire world. During an April 23 Coronavirus Task Force briefing, Bill Bryan from the Department of Homeland Security stated that laboratory research indicated that "The virus dies quickest in sunlight." This led the President to ask Bryan, "So supposing we hit the body with a tremendous — whether it's ultraviolet or just a very powerful light—supposing you brought the light inside the body, which you can do either through the skin or some other way."

No one dared question his Dr. Hans Zarkov line of thought. Someone should have stood up and yelled "Mr. President, you must be crazy!" but such an intuitive response was not forthcoming. The floodgates opened wider when the President added more extemporaneous hypothesizing, stating "I see the disinfectant that knocks it out in a minute, one minute. And is there a way we can do something like that by injection inside or almost a cleaning? As you see, it gets in the lungs, it does a tremendous number on the lungs, so it would be interesting to check that."

Scientist and doctors at Johns Hopkins Medicine were eager to "check that" suggestion; the unanimous conclusion probably dumbfounded the President. Regarding the Trump misinformation about the swallowing, injecting or topically applying bleach and various disinfectants, Johns Hopkins Medicine stated, "These products are highly toxic and should *never* be swallowed or injected into the body. Call 911 if this occurs. Disinfectants, bleach and soap and water may be used to clean surfaces, an important prevention step in stopping the spread of coronavirus and COVID-19...**Never** attempt to self-treat or prevent COVID-19 by rubbing or bathing with bleach, disinfectants, or rubbing alcohol anywhere on your body."[35]

Health authorities across the globe unanimously decried the notion. One such statement read, "It should go without saying that this idea is dangerously, mind-bogglingly wrong, but apparently these truths are no longer self-evident in 2020. So I will reiterate in the strongest of terms: ***do not, under any circumstances, inject, drink, or otherwise introduce bleach or any other disinfectant into your body.*** The corrosive substance will burn your insides, may permanently damage your organs, and could even kill you. It will also be incredibly painful the entire time you are dying."[36]

Our mercurial President dialed back his words the next day, claiming he was speaking "sarcastically to reporters like you, just to see what would happen." Instead of apologizing for making this dangerously idiotic remark, he dug himself deeper into a hole, using a defense which any clear-thinking person would immediately categorize as problematic.

In the first place, President Trump does not test reporters' gullibility. He reacts to what they say by calling it fake news. Second, if he had expected reporters to follow him down the primrose path, he should not have insulted them. Third, his lame excuse would have been more successful and considerably more entertaining if he had quoted Mel Brooks' Young Frankenstein. When Victor Frankenstein attempted to talk his way out of the cell within which he was confined with his monster, he yelled to Igor and Inga, "What's the matter with you people? I was joking! Don't you know a joke when you hear one? HA-HA-HA-HA!" We knew that both Victor and Donald were liars, but at the very least, Victor was not being "sarcastic" in acknowledging his folly.

That disinfectant "joke" reverberated throughout the Northeast corridor and across the nation, but no one was laughing. Officials manning 911 calls on April 24 were swamped with inquiries about injecting disinfectants. For example, a spokesperson for Maryland's Governor Larry Hogan described how his state's Emergency Management team received "more than 100 calls"[37] leading them to post a notice about the dangers of using disinfectants. In New York, "18 hours after Trump's comments, the Poison Center received 30 exposure calls about disinfectants. Ten involved bleach, 9 were about Lysol, and 11 others regarding other household cleaners. Compared to the same time window last year, there were a total of 13 exposure calls, with 2 involving bleach, but none involving Lysol-type products."[38] Calls to Illinois' Poison Control Center spiked on April 24, culminating in a call from "another individual who gargled with a mixture of mouthwash and bleach intended to kill the coronavirus."[39]

Parents who thought that soaking their children's hands with sanitizers would safeguard those youngsters from the Coronavirus did not realize three things: first, that "The amount of alcohol in hand sanitizer ranges from 40% to 95%. Most hand sanitizer products contain over 60% ethyl alcohol, a stronger alcohol concentration than most hard liquors:" second, that **"Even a small amount of alcohol can cause alcohol poisoning in**

children. Alcohol poisoning can cause confusion, vomiting and drowsiness, and in severe cases, respiratory arrest and death;" and third, children are prone to putting their hands in their mouths when parents are not looking. Consequently, by April 30, poison control centers in the United States managed an aggregate of "7,593 exposure cases about hand sanitizer in children 12 years and younger."[40]

The White House tried once more to employ a "he was only joking" defense to derail an inauspicious Trumpism voiced during his speech at his Tulsa, Oklahoma rally on June 20. President Trump downplayed the importance of national testing, implying there was no cause for alarm. More testing, he claimed, meant there would be more positive cases. To decrease this number of positive cases, a number which he believed to be artificially inflated, he recommended that the United States reduce the number of tests given to its citizens.

The six thousand, two hundred fans of the President who were stupid enough to attend the rally and dumb enough not to wear masks, cheered the President's suggestion to lessen the number of tests Americans should receive. The rest of the nation was dumbfounded by President Trump's errant remark about reducing the number of COVID-19 tests being given, but not the Trump attendees, who had waited for days to enjoy the rally. Whether they stood next to each other on the Center's floor for nearly six hours, or filled the first-balcony seats that represented a quarter of the BOK Center's nineteen thousand seats, they had decided to treasure each passing moment of the super-spreader event.

These revelers wholeheartedly supported the belief that testing imposed a restriction on their personal freedom. They also extolled an outlandish warning issued by the President, who asserted, "If the Democrats gain power, then the rioters will be in charge." He told the witlessly gullible crowd that if he was not re-elected, "Your 401-K's will be worthless."

President Trump elicited from the crowd the same fervor that characterized the NSDAP Nuremberg rally of 1936. President Trump threw down the gauntlet to his supporters at the BOK Center and those watching the rally on Fox News by reminding them of the inchoate power they possessed. To meet his goal of suppressing Radical Left Anarchists, Agitators, and Looters, he told the nation, "If our people were violent, it would be a terrible, terrible day for the other side." This was no joke; if things had gone differently in the streets of Tulsa after the rally that night, his statement could have been construed as an incitement to riot.

Fortunately, the attendees were too tired after waiting, applauding, and screaming for so many hours at the BOK Center. They dispersed without incident, adjourning to mix it up with the yahoos at the Mercury Lounge, the Valkyrie, the Soundpony, and the Colony bars, sharing Jello shots while hollering at each other and applauding the raucous performances of the Blue Water Highway Band and the Dirty River Boys with Cotton James at the Mercury.

On June 21, White House spokespersons deflected the import of the President's nasty suggestions, claiming the President was "joking" abut limiting the number of tests given and bragging about the power his supporters would embody if they turned violent. Later that day, when asked by a reporter if he was indeed "joking," President Trump told her "I never kid." He must have forgotten that on April 24 he claimed that when he made his remark about injecting disinfectants he was only joking.

The glib statements the President made in Tulsa echoed the nonsensical sentiments he had expressed at each of his Coronavirus Task Force briefings. It was easy for him to escape repercussions from outlandish claims made at a rally, but it was more difficult for him to walk away unscathed when he opened his mouth in the presence of a group of reporters who would rightly question the veracity of each of his statements. His ability to play to the camera and to doubletalk his way out of what he believed to be an unfair interrogation had become strained. Once President Trump was convinced that damage incurred by the outrageous ad hoc statements he would make in future briefings far outweighed any political cache that he might accrue by continuing to hold nightly court in the Brady Room, the briefings ended with a whimper.

President Trump stymied the dissemination of real information by discontinuing these daily televised briefings. In doing so, he punished the American public and undermined the efforts of newspaper and television reporters to relay to us new facts about the Coronavirus pandemic. His action represented a comeuppance to the reporters whom he considered to be enemies of the people.

The cessation of the Task Force Briefings was our contemporary equivalent of the 1933 raid on the offices of the <u>Munich Post</u> by the Chancellor of Germany. Reporters who asked hard questions at the Task Force Briefings had been defamed as "bad, very bad" people, "terrible" people who had the temerity to ask "nasty" questions. President Trump handled Weijia Jiang, Peter Alexander, Yamiche Alcindor, and Kaitlan Collins with the same wantonness that Martin Gruber, Erhard Auer, Edmund Goldschagg, and Julius Zerfass had experienced, courtesy of their Chancellor.

The abrupt end of the Briefings provided another example of the President's ongoing policy of containment—not containment of the Coronavirus pandemic, but containment of all sources of news that could cause the President political damage. Dr. Bright had been fired, Inspectors General lost jobs, the Ft. Detrick recommendations were thrown in the Presidential shredder, the CDC was muzzled, funding for the World Health Organization was withdrawn, Dr. Birx's "core elements of a testing plan," consisting of "robust diagnostic testing," "timely monitoring systems for new cases," and a "rapid-response program" were never implemented, the fifteen-day plan to arrest the spread of the Coronavirus ended fifteen days after the paper plan was introduced, and Dr. Fauci's warnings to Congress were dismissed with a Presidential wave of a hand and with a snide comment by the President that Dr. Fauci "wants to play it both ways."

The American public was expected to take the President's statements at face value and express undying gratitude to him for doing such a Great Job. We were to thank him for not starting a nuclear war with North Korea because "if anyone else," by which he meant former Secretary of State Hillary Clinton, "had been President we would be at war right now." During the Cuban Missile Crisis, President Kennedy never said, "if Richard Nixon had been President, we would be at war with Russia," even though that assessment would most likely have been accurate.

President Trump's dereliction of his duty to the citizens of America could not be contained. The strutting egoist at center stage continued to flaunt his churlish wares. It is a guilt-edged certainty that Mr. Trump believes he can say or do whatever he wants because he is the President, forgetting that he is bound by the Constitution to safeguard, not endanger American lives. He forsakes that oath each time he puts his political interests ahead of his duty to preserve and protect; he plays Faustus when we need him to be like Fauci.

Americans are smart, brave, and innovative. I know that our courage and resilience will see us through the autocratic strong-arming we receive from the powers that be. Rock musicians like Neil Young, who songs express a social consciousness, have traditionally upheld the belief that their songs are platforms from which their voices of dissent can be heard. When thinking about President Trump's bending of the truth to suit his purposes, I was reminded of a song by Muse called "Uprising." The lyrics espoused the same alternate view of society that rang true and clear in the Sixties. In the best tradition of Jefferson Airplane's "We Can Be Together," Muse sang,

> They'll try to push drugs
> That keep us all dumbed down and hope that
> We will never see the truth around
>
> They will not force us
> They will stop degrading us
> They will not control us
> We will be victorious

We are not mice running in a maze from which only the President of the United States knows how to escape. He is not a doctor, though he views himself as being better informed than most doctors. He is not a scientist, but he believes he knows more than scientists currently studying the Coronavirus. He is not a lawyer, though he believes he can nominate "perfect" court justices.

We can look behind the curtain and ignore the garbled mess of rhetoric with which we are assaulted every day. I know that we can act to preserve our lives and well-being and we will be victorious, no thanks to the madman who does not know the meaning of Federalism. He can proclaim the country open; we can stay at home and be safe. By following that prudent course of action, we can limit the spread of the Coronavirus which means, as Pearl Jam sang, we will still be alive.

I dozed through the rest of March 31 and slept fitfully that night. One of the items not included in the "Symptoms" section of my handout was **"Expect to have the strangest dreams of your life."** My dreams were not always scary, but what I discovered when recalling those dreams in the light of day was frightening. Most of my dreams featured the presence of departed friends of mine, my parents, and relatives returning to communicate with me. I wondered if this meant I would be soon joining them in the Hereafter.

I had never been preoccupied with death, and now suddenly it was in the forefront of my subconscious. I did not particularly want to dream about my own death or the people I had known who were deceased. I would have preferred my feverish imagination to conjure spicy images of Anna Torv, Vera Farmiga, Mary McCormack, Michelle Phillips, Mary Louise Parker, Tea Leoni, Ashley Judd, Maria Bello, and Salma Hayek. But no, instead of allowing me to have those far more pleasant dreams, COVID-19 had created for me the dream-state persona of Dr. Malcolm Crowe, the psychologist who saw dead people.

At about noon I felt levelheaded enough to walk to my kitchen, sit at my table, take my temperature, pulse, and blood pressure, and record the results in my Abbey Road notebook. I made a pot of green tea and listed the things I needed to do that day to feel better. I knew what "remedies" to avoid, and my record of symptoms and measurements would indicate what I needed to fix.

Lists were an essential weapon in my battle to survive COVID-19, because if I could focus my mental activities long enough to make a list of everything I needed to remember to do that day, I would not spend hours trying to recall any one item in the plan that may have escaped my purview. Making a list provided me with a sense of accomplishment and with renewed confidence that I had a plan in place. My approach was multi-faceted; since my symptoms were intermittent, it made sense that no single, decorous solution would lead me to recovery.

I did not include Hallmark generalities like "Start feeling better!" I wanted to make each specific item in my plan easily attainable. The list that I had been developing included about twenty common-sense reminders, for instance, to turn off electrical appliance after using, to feed the cat and clean out the litterbox, to walk slowly when going downstairs to pick up the mail or take out the trash, and to check my phone occasionally for any texts. That morning I added the following five goals, based on two assumptions: that I would test positive for COVID-19, and that some form of proactive engagement might help me recover. My new additions were:

- Find out everything I can about what the Coronavirus does to my immune system once infection occurs

- Determine what physical actions and exercises might help me recover

- Decide which vitamins and supplements I could safely take to aid the recovery process

- Generate a similar list of foods that will help with recovery

- Wait until I feel alert to go to grocery and drug stores to purchase all required items

What I had learned about the Coronavirus from watching <u>MSNBC</u> for several hours each day was that the once Coronavirus settles in my lungs, my immune system reacts with a mechanism called a cytokine storm. I googled the term and found that it was defined as "A severe immune reaction in which the body releases too many cytokines into the blood too quickly. Cytokines play an important role in normal immune responses but having a large amount of them released in the body all at once can be harmful. A cytokine storm can occur as a result of an infection, auto-immune condition, or other disease. It may also occur after treatment with some types of immunotherapy. Signs and symptoms include high fever, inflammation (redness and swelling), and severe fatigue and nausea. Sometimes, a cytokine storm may be severe or life threatening and lead to multiple organ failure."[41]

To put that formidable description in as unscientific terms as possible, once the a virus finds a home in my lungs and acclimates itself to its new environment, my immune system recognizes the virus as an unwanted intruder, a squatter moving into prime real estate. Eager to usurp the landowners property and claim it as its breeding grounds, the Coronavirus stands its ground. My immune system properly calls in local authorities, the cytokines, to kick out the squatter. But my immune system goes too far and orders the equivalent of a tactical nuclear strike. The fallout from the overabundant supply of cytokines is widespread and contaminates my lungs and nearby organs such as my heart and liver. The storm's fibrotic effect on my lungs has been called Covid Pneumonia, which is the one of the bad results of a Coronavirus infection.

I recognized that this storm would pose a serious risk to my life. I had read once that keeping my lungs moist was an effective measure against pneumonia, which seemed odd, because pneumonia is often defined by a buildup of fluids in the lungs. I wondered if such a counterintuitive measure could work for treating COVID-19.

I recalled a scene in <u>World War Z</u> when, just before Dr. Fassbach dies, he provides Gerry Lane with this metaphor: "Mother Nature is a serial killer. No one's better, more creative. But like all serial killers, she can't help the urge to want to get caught. And what good are all those brilliant crimes if no one takes the credit? So she leaves crumbs. Now the hard part, why you spend a decade in school, is seeing the crumbs for the clues they are. Sometimes the thing you thought was the most brutal aspect of the virus turns out to be the chink in its armor. And she loves disguising her weaknesses as strengths."

Right or wrong, I decided to apply the logic of this fictional work to my real-life situation. I was coughing nearly all the time, and I wondered if I could safely add small amounts of moisture to my lungs which I guessed were in a pre-Covid Pneumonia stage. I could do that on a regular basis by inhaling steam from the pot of green tea while it brewed. I could also spend a few minutes several times a day inhaling while holding a hot, damp washcloth against my face. I would exhale against the pressure of the washcloth, which I hoped would result in my longs becoming stronger and more pliant.

I applied the same bread crumb logic to another worrisome symptom. My temperatures were intermittent, ranging from one hundred and one to one hundred and three, and I had been using aspirin every four hours to reduce it by a few degrees. Perhaps the Coronavirus could not survive in my lungs at a higher internal temperature. I was confident I could tolerate a fever as high as one hundred three for a while without inducing hyperthermia. If *not* taking aspirin and letting my fever rage for a few hours worked, I would have used COVID-19's strength to cause a fever to degrade its ability to kill me. I was aware that not everyone would agree with my concept of using the plot of a zombie movie to treat COVID-19, so I did not share my planned approach with anyone at the time.

I employed a more conventional protocol to settle on which therapeutic actions, which exercises would help improve my condition. I had been in the habit of running long distances three times a week before I became ill, and I thought jogging for short distances each day would help strengthen my lungs. There were two reasons why I listed that activity as possible but perhaps not a good idea: first, it would require a sizeable amount of will power to force myself to jog when I viewed getting out of bed as a herculean task; second, it would not be good to collapse on the road because, instead of strengthening my cardio-vascular system, I had overtaxing my already-weakened lungs. I needed to devote more thought to this item before I laced my Nikes and had a go at it.

Because I was spending so much time twisting and turning while in a prone position while I tried unsuccessfully to find a comfortable way to sleep, I concluded that unless I acted now to prevent it, in a week's time, maybe less, I would pull muscles in my back, stomach, and sides out of whack. I decided to start doing sit-ups each day. I would begin trying to do twenty-five, and if that worked, I would increase by ten each day until I maxed out at two hundred a day. I felt a naturel disinclination to perform any act resembling exercising when my head felt as though it was split lengthwise down the middle, throbbing in the back, and pounding in the front like the drumbeat in Led Zeppelin's "When the Levee Breaks."

I never viewed myself as an abstemious person, but because I had no appetite, I was skipping meals. It was an omission which resulted in me having no energy to anything more strenuous than channel surfing. I committed myself to eating more food than I felt like swallowing. Breakfast had consisted of toast and green tea. I would add oatmeal and raisins to that meal. In the afternoon, I would eat a handful of olives and a thick slice of Cambozola Black Label cheese. Two weeks prior I had spent ninety dollars purchasing a five-pound wheel of the stuff at Igourmet, figuring it would last a while. The strong flavor of the creamy cheese registered dimly on my depleted taste buds. I decided I would eat crackers with the cheese each afternoon, and I would double the amount of cheese that I consumed.

I understood that to accomplish my meager form of sit-up exercises with some degree of success, I would need to attain a caloric state of homeostasis, which meant adding carbs at dinner time. I decided to eat pasta every night. I planned to cook a gallon of tomato sauce using sauce, paste, basil, oregano, crushed tomatoes, some red wine, a tablespoon of sugar, omitting garlic. I would alternate marinara pasta meals with ones adorned with olive oil and parmesan. I would in effect transform myself into a customer at an Olive Garden Restaurant, devouring my bottomless entrée each night, but unlike that diner, I would not suffer from food poisoning two hours after I concluded my meal. I would not be able to smell my marinara sauce as it simmered, but I remembered its scent and taste from the years that my Italian grandmother, my aunts, and my mother made their marinara, and that memory would suffice.

I realized that the process of doing sit ups on my yoga mat would be a boring, depressing, and painful. I needed to maintain a positive attitude about exercising, and I decided that if I added music to the routine, time would pass a little more quickly and pleasantly.

I had lived my entire life with vinyl. I made a slow transition to compact discs in the Eighties when Born in the USA and Brothers in Arms were first released, but that is where I drew the line. I had no music on my phone and no Ipod with play-rotation capability. I decided to use songs from a select set of cds instead of playing vinyl albums during my workout. I had a six-cd player with a remote control, which made it easy to toggle between selections as I gasped for breath. I estimated that I would spend ten to fifteen minutes exercising each day, and I would need to play at least two lengthy songs consecutively. The music had to be rhythmically and thematically appropriate. I selected three songs that qualified on both fronts: "Do You Feel Like We Do" from Frampton Comes Alive, Thunderclap Newman's "Something in the Air," and the first three tracks of Green Day's 21st Century Breakdown.

I treated Sonia's "incurable" disease by placing it within a context that I understood. Emulating that process, I spent some time researching the pros and cons of various vitamins and minerals. I augmented the limited approach I used to treat a cold by including different supplements that might positively affect the periphery and core of my symptoms. Many of the items were water soluble, but some were fat-soluble, so I needed to eat a fat-containing food each time I took my vitamins and supplements.

I decided it would be safe and possibly helpful to take the following pills each morning:

- B complex with 2.5mg Thiamin, 2.5mg Riboflavin, 5mg Niacin, 100mcg B-12, and 10mg Protease

- 1,000mg of Vitamin C with rose hips and a bioflavinoid complex

- 50mcg of D3-2000

- 400IU of Vitamin E (as di-alpha tocopheryl, not tocopheryl acetate)

- A men's 50+ Multivitamin

- Acidophilus

- 2,800mg of Fish Oil in each of 2 softgels to total 1,960mg of Omega-3

- 1,00mg of L-Arginine

- 1 gram of L-Lysine

- 15mg of Lycopene

- 160mg of Saw Palmetto

I would take an additional 1,000mg of Vitamin C pill every four hours. Each evening I would take all the above plus twenty-five milligrams of Chelated Zinc. Instead of taking a Men's multivitamin, Lycopene, and Saw Palmetto, I suppose that women would require a Women's multivitamin, four hundred micrograms of Folic Acid, and three hundred milligrams of St. John's Wort three times a day.

I wanted to consume some version of a smoothie each morning. I did not think that Rocky Balboa's predawn libation of six raw eggs would be helpful, but the concept of an emulsified drink rich in protein, healthy fats, and vegetables was appealing. I had purchased a "Ninja Auto IQ Nutri-Ninja Blender Duo" at a garage sale in October 2019, but I had not touched it after testing the huge chrome and plastic contraption to verify that it worked. It had come with a booklet of various recipes.

After researching the variety of possible ingredients suggested in the Ninja cookbook, I made an uneducated determination of which ones would be optimal for fighting COVID-19. I then estimated the maximum quantity of each ingredient that would fit into the Ninja's plastic container. I felt that the following food items would effective and palatable:

- 4 average size leaves of deveined, organic romaine

- 42 almonds

- 1 large organic carrot cut into one-inch pieces

- 1 large stalk of organic celery similarly cut

- 2 tablespoons of organic flaxseed meal

- 1/2 teaspoon of turmeric

- 1/4 teaspoon of ground black pepper

- 1 banana

- 24 ounces of apple juice

I avoided including vegetables like broccoli, cauliflower, asparagus, and green beans for two reasons: first, I would prefer to eat them with dinner; and second, I was not sure what would happen to the consistency of my mixture if I add that much more bulk.

Once I placed the above items into the Ninja's storage tank, I would fill it with all the apple juice that would fit, being careful not to exceed the

Ninja container's thirty-two-ounce capacity. I could tinker with the above formula, and I could adjust it as my condition deteriorated or improved, but I felt confident I had arrived at a workable core solution. Before doing anything else though, I heated my Chick Fil-A sandwich, ate it, and took a nap. It was already 4 p.m. and I was tired.

Feeling refreshed and alert after an hour of dozing, armed with my Amex card and my list, I drove cautiously to Jewel's, Trader Joe's, Whole Foods, Walgreens, and CVS to purchase what I needed. I procured a supply of other essentials items such as grapefruit juice, ten pounds of assorted pasta, sourdough bread, crystallized ginger, two three-liter cans of Artemis First Cold Pressing Extra Virgin olive oil, Gatorade, six gallons of apple juice, a case of Diet Cherry Coke, pretzels, cookies, and Butterfingers bars.

At CVS, which was my final stop, I purchased another digital oral thermometer. I saw the new touchless type, but old habits die hard. I would have preferred glass and mercury thermometers because no battery is required, but they are dangerous when held with a shaky hand and placed between chattering teeth under a sore tongue. I did not want to find myself touching broken glass, or touching, breathing, or swallowing mercury in the middle of the night. I noticed a display of pulse oximeters, but since I did not know at the time that this item would turn out to be a crucial piece of equipment for me to have on hand, one which would soon be sold out of every drug store, medical supplies store, and hospital pharmacy in the greater Chicagoland area, I did not purchase one.

After I arrived home and refrigerated most of my purchases, I took a low dose aspirin and eighty milligrams of Atorvastatin. Before I crashed, I showered and fed Sonia, who had indicated to me that it was past time for her Turkey Delight dinner. I was cold and exhausted, and I forego a pasta evening. Instead I ate a Butterfingers bar and drank a glass of Gatorade.

The next morning, I took my five milligrams of Lisinopril, but I skipped the forty milligrams of Omeprazole that I had been taking because I had not eaten enough to warrant a dose. I started my sit up regimen. After twenty-five laboriously slow sit ups, I stopped. I was sweating and breathing heavily. I had not expected to feel chipper during or after this initial set of exercises, but I was happy to have started. I was confident that, next out of the gate, I would reach the number thirty-five before I collapsed on my mat.

I struggled to my feet, ambled into the kitchen, and began to prepare my Ninja eye-opener. Romaine is the best lettuce for hydrating and is the most easily digestible type. The almonds and flaxseed were my source of protein. Almonds are the healthiest of nuts, and forty-two was the exact number specified as optimal for an adult. If I could have fit more than one carrot into the Ninja container I would have done so; raw carrots are healthier than cooked ones. The flaxseed meal was an additional protein source, one that is high in omega threes. Turmeric possesses anti-inflammatory properties. It is found in curry, a spice blend which improves cardiovascular functioning and has an abundance of antioxidant properties. Black pepper is needed to allow the body to absorb turmeric. My mother was a proponent of the saying "An apple a day keeps the doctor away," and the amount of apple juice in my concoction was the equivalent of several kilos of Fuji apples.

After I had completed the required rinsing, slicing, and measuring and had crammed all of it into the container, I added the apple juice, sealed the top, placed the inverted container into the body of the machine, and pushed the proper buttons to allow the Ninja perform its twenty-second pulse, low, medium, and high cycle. I hoped my Big Gulp would have a viscosity somewhere between tap water and the type of sludge I would get if I acquired a cup of liquid from the Chicago Sanitary and Ship Canal. The resulting emulsification that morning was a bit thicker than I thought it would be, but otherwise it seemed like I could drink it without choking. Its color resembled that of the sand at Indiana Dunes State Park. If I wanted a greener appearance, I would need either to add more romaine or to use less turmeric.

I had prepared a week's supply of my vitamins and supplements in my pill container which had morning and evening compartments. This time-saving tool also provided me with an easy way to verify that I had remembered to take the day's proper allotment. Although it might seem that disremembering such a mundane chore is an early sign of Alzheimer's, I can assure you that when caught in the grip of COVID-19, simple tasks become much more difficult to perform in a reliable manner.

I likened my mental condition in these weeks to how I would feel after consuming five shots of Crown Royal or too many milligrams of edible cannabis, except I did not feel euphoric. I felt miserable. I experienced a stumbling-drunk level of frustration over my inefficient thoughts and meandering actions. My frustration was heightened by the realization that my problems were not caused by a drug such as alcohol or cannabis. Those debilitating symptoms would wear off in six to eight hours, as the potency of the specific drug declined. My timeframe for release from COVID-19 inebriation would be six to eight weeks.

In the meantime, it would take a great deal of effort to clear every muddled thought, to avoid every pitfall that I might encounter on an average day. The last time I utilized such a concerted effort of concentration to focus on small details while remembering the large picture was forty years ago, at my Ph.D. dissertation defense. This time, instead of being intellectually ambushed when I was asked to explain out of the blue T.S. Elliott's objective correlative criticism of <u>Hamlet</u>, I was being emotionally and physically assaulted by a COVID-19 battering ram.

The quantity of pills and gels I needed to take each morning and evening was a bit scary, but I could not eliminate any of them to make the mass easier to swallow. My B-complex and multivitamin were required to meet and exceed the RDA. Vitamin C was an essential component. Nobel Prize-winning chemist Dr. Linus Pauling believed in its curative effects, and I found his words to be a compelling endorsement. The D3 vitamin seemed to be an insignificantly small softgel but it packed a wallop for preventing heart disease. I began taking it when lived near Seattle, where time spent outdoors in sunlight is limited, and I have been taking it ever since.

I thought Vitamin E would strengthen my immune system, which was surely impacted by the Coronavirus. I did not know what the Coronavirus would do to my digestive tract, so I took Acidophilus to protect gastrointestinal bacteria functionality. The Omega-3 fish oil megadose would raise my high-density lipid level, which I hoped would counteract all the Cambozola cheese I would be eating.

L-Lysine was shown to be helpful for reducing stress; it also possessed antiviral properties. I believed it was helping Sonia stay alive. I was aware that what worked for a cat might not work well for a human, but desperate times call for desperate measures, which in this case meant thinking out-side the box of rationality. The lycopene, saw palmetto, and evening dose of zinc would hopefully raise my testosterone level. This left one supplement in which was putting a great deal of stock, L-Arginine.

I knew that the hydrochloride component of L-Arginine was thought to help boost concentration and improve circulation, but I had different, perhaps farfetched reason to include it. I have watched by my count ten thousand movies in my life. Film study was my area of interest. It was the subject of my dissertation and my first book. I learned much about life from movies. Films provided me with a unique ontological perspective, and they were my primary referent when I tackled real-life problems. Which brought me directly back to my <u>Andromeda Strain</u> speculations.

Once Peter Jackson had been examined in the Andromeda BSL-4 facility, tests results showed that he was an alcoholic who had survived the Andromeda virus by drinking Squeeze, a nickname for the canned heat called Sterno. It raised the level of acidity in his bloodstream, and consequently held the Andromeda virus in abeyance. I could not drink Sterno twice a day to survive the Coronavirus; if I did, I would never get a good night's sleep, and the cure would be worse than the disease. There was also no room left in my thirty-two-ounce Ninja container for a Sterno additive.

L-Arginine is the amino acid that the body converts into nitric oxide. I had learned that the Coronavirus can exist in water, even if the water had varying, that is higher levels of acidity. All right, I thought, maybe it can live in water of higher acidity, but I asked myself, can it also live comfortably in my body if my system is more acidic than the environment of other human Coronavirus hosts? I was not confident that drinking grapefruit juice and taking vitamin C would sufficiently raise my bloodstream's acidity high enough to accomplish my goal of staying alive. Research indicated that it was safe to take two to six grams of L-Arginine per day, so I was comfortable starting with my two grams, in the sincere hope that my Coronavirus would view the approaching nitric oxide with the same trepidation I would feel if someone forced me to stick the tines of a fork into a two hundred and twenty volt electrical outlet.

I decided not to take my Omeprazole capsule, which would have decreased my system's acidity. I had a supply of drugs that had been prescribed for me to treat CIDP pain, anxiety, depression, sleeplessness, and seizures. These included bacoflen, gabapentin, fluoxetine, trazadone, hydrocodone, and oxycodone. I could not find any research indicating that those heavy-duty meds would disable the Coronavirus. The few times I was given those drugs in the hospital, they had an alarmingly disabling effect on me. I thought that taking any of those now would be akin to lighting a match while standing inside a dynamite shack. Also, I did not require a more befuddled frame of mind, which would be the result of taking anyone of those six drugs. The Coronavirus served adequately to confound my thought processes, impede my physical dexterity, and disrupt my emotional equilibrium.

To avoid taking hydrocodone when I lived in Washington state, I used legal, recreational marijuana with fourteen to one levels of CBD vs. THC to treat the pain. When I returned to Illinois, I applied for and received a medical cannabis pilot program card. As was the case with all alternative forms of Coronavirus therapies, the jury was still out on the role cannabis might play in the battle against COVID-19. I decided not to use flowers which would have had a deleterious effect on my breathing capacity. I would also avoid using edibles which would heighten my lack of ability to focus and might induce a higher degree of paranoia about my medical condition. My life would be enough of a chemistry experiment without adding those uncertainties into the mix. I was sure that my home-cooked regimen of vitamins, supplements, and nutrients could be safely included in my daily routine. My only uncertainty involved was how to swallow the handful of pills and softgels without choking.

It took a while for me in my present condition to work out a solution to a problem which a few weeks ago would have been a no-brainer. I stared at the pile of pills, forgetting the intent and purpose of the reliable warhorse—Cartesian logic—which I was attempting to apply to solve the too-many-pill problem I faced. One moment I was convinced that I could swallow more pills at one time than humanly possible. The next moment I saw myself collapsed on the floor, choking on too many pills, with no EMT nearby to perform a Heimlich Maneuver and save my life. I did not realize at the time that this was the degree to which COVID-19 had short-circuited mental faculties that I like to believe were otherwise acute. I thought my confusion was due to ambient stress, not realizing that the stress I was experiencing was COVID-19-induced. I contemplated increasing my dosage of L-Lysine, but I did not want to suffer digestive distress or kidney damage. I was sure a solution was hidden nearby, and with the right set of eyes I would discern its location. I took as deep of a breath as I was capable, checked my blood pressure which was now one-sixty over one-ten, and tried to consider my options calmly.

A eureka moment occurred five minutes into my internal debate, when I realized that I could avert any unpleasantness by only putting a portion of that morning's allotment in my mouth at any given time. I reduced the number of pills in my hand by fifty percent. Imagining that I was eating a chocolate croissant while sipping on a robustly sweetened cappuccino, I swallowed half the pills with first my quaff of the mixture. I held the container with one hand when I drank it, though I later learned from the President that using a two-handed approach to drinking was the surefire way to keep me from spilling the liquid on my long, red necktie, if I had one that matched my orange and blue pajamas.

The morning melange went down easily and was not as unpleasant as I had feared, thanks to taste buds that no longer functioned properly. There was no context within which the word "smoothie" could be applied to this concoction, which had a coffee-grounds consistency. I would not have been able to pour it down my throat if I had not included so much apple juice. It took about twenty minutes to drink the entire quart of the amalgam.

Although I was no longer in a mood for more imbibing, I drank three cups of green tea. It was an essential component in my fight with the Coronavirus. Its benefits ranged from cancer prevention to increasing memory functions. Its curative effects have been studied throughout the world. The goal of the renowned biochemist and green tea drinker Shutsung Liao was "to put science into herbal medicine, to investigate the molecular actions of herbal medicines and to study novel approaches to therapies."[42] He conducted a University of Chicago study and found that one of green tea's compounds, epigallocatechin gallate, worked "to inhibit the growth of certain tumors." If it worked for cancer prevention, it might trounce the Coronavirus, and if there was any chance of it helping me remember to pay my Comcast internet bill on time, I would gladly drink as much of the bitter tea of Dr. Liao as I could each morning.

I found that inhaling its steam through my mouth was the safer way to proceed. If the steam seemed too hot on my lips, it would be too hot for my lungs. I kept my head ten to twelve inches above the water level in the half-gallon pot I was using to brew the tea. To help absorb some to the massive amount of liquid that had hit my stomach, I ate two slices of sour dough toast with my bowl of brown sugar and raisin oatmeal.

The entire breakfast process took about an hour to complete, which I hoped was time well spent. Four hours later, the fluids had sufficiently flushed my system. My efforts would not wash away the Coronavirus, but I hoped that would help me fight its ill-effects. My stomach was mildly upset by this liquid assault, a side effect easily mollified by a single berry-flavored, ultra-strength antacid.

I had been more active the past two days than I had the entire previous week, and by noon, the expenditure of energy had taken its toll. My headache had returned with a vengeance. I rested for a while and watched television before I picked up my acoustic guitar and practiced. Incessant coughing had changed my singing voice, and I no longer had trouble with the baritone lines of "Cold Jordan" which was the song I played that afternoon. Jerry Garcia favored that traditional spiritual song when he jammed with New Riders of the Purple Sage. I could only manage one, maybe two songs on a good day, because sitting up or standing exacerbated my urge to cough, and I could not play or sing while sprawled on my back. I remember Dean Martin singing "My Riffle, My Pony, and Me" while reclining on his jail cell cot in <u>Rio Bravo</u>, but that is not an easy task to accomplish.

I was fortunate that I did not have any airline ticketing chores to accomplish, because I could not have functioned efficiently. I had no energy or inclination to eat dinner or take vitamins that night, and by 8 p.m. I was ready to sleep. To take my mind off my aching body, I let my thoughts wander. I contemplated questions for the ages. Were the Beatles renaissance minstrels in previous lives, as Fabio Traverso imagined them to be? Did Van Halen's cover of "You Really Got Me" compare favorably to the Kink's original release? If Blue Oyster Cult could have played at Woodstock, would their song have been called "Don't Fear the Reefer?" Did people named James purchase more GMC Jimmy vehicles than people named Joe or Mary?

I fell asleep quickly, but the night became truly frightening. I awoke at 214 a.m. on April 3 experiencing a severe shortness of breath. Although that term sounds like an ordinary, run of the mill inconvenience and not something to ruffle one's feathers, the next two hours were scarier than I had thought likely or possible.

I did not wake up because I was breathing more rapidly. I woke up in a panic because breathing ceased to be an autonomic reflex. I was alarmed to discover that when I kept perfectly still, resting on my back, my normal pattern of taking a breath every two seconds was no longer happening. I gasped and sat up in bed, and consciously took a breath every two seconds. I continued to force myself to breathe for a minute or two, and then I stopped and waited to see if my normal breathing pattern would return. It did not. I thought that sitting up in a chair would kick start the process, but I found that I still had to concentrate on each inhalation and exhalation to make them happen.

When I realized I could not breathe, I flashed back to event that had occurred many years ago. I am certified for Advanced Open Water Diving by the Professional Association of Diving Instructors. One day while I was on a familiarization trip to Club Med in Bora Bora, I went on a patch reef dive near Miri Miri.

When diving in unfamiliar territory, a buddy system is utilized. Fifteen minutes into the dive I had seventy percent of my air remaining, and I decided it was time to return to the dive boat. My buddy had not been checking his supply of air. He had also failed to check his supply when he started the dive, which is a mistake never made by a responsible diver. While I was at seventy percent, he was at fifteen percent.

We were about ten minutes from the dive boat, and I knew he would never make it back to the boat before his supply was exhausted. We could not surface and swim using our snorkels, because I could see a barracuda if I were forty feet underwater, and I could swim away from it. I would not be able to see a barracuda approaching if I were swimming on the surface, and I guessed that my buddy, who was already panicking, would not survive a surface swim.

I signaled him to stay with me, and we began sharing my air. The protocol to follow when in that predicament is for me to take two deep breaths, hand my mouthpiece to my buddy, who in theory would take two breaths and return it to me, and we would repeat the process as often as necessary. To my surprise, when I handed my mouthpiece to him, he did not reciprocate after taking his two breaths. I ran out of breath, but I did not panic. I tapped him on his facemask and using the Donald Trump two-handed approach, I jerked my mouthpiece out of his mouth. He had nearly chewed off the bite tabs, but I could seal the piece with my lips.

After two breaths, I removed it, held it while pushed it into his mouth for two breaths, pulled it out, and I continued in that manner until we reached the dive boat, at which point I had five percent of my air remaining. Both myself and the divemaster had a serious discussion with the gentleman who was my buddy. To my knowledge, he never dove again in Bora Bora waters.

I realized on the morning of April 3 that what was happening to me was not good. It felt horrible not to be able to breathe—it was as though someone neglected to give my mouthpiece back to me. I was afraid that if I went to sleep, I might not be able to wake in time to begin breathing.

Another striking comparison from my past occurred to me as I consciously forced myself to breathe. When I was in my running prime in the 1980s, I would often push myself to an extreme when running a ten-kilometer cross-country event. I completed one of those races in under thirty minutes, and at its conclusion, I could not catch my breath. Although I was breathing as hard as I could, I could not intake sufficient air to slow my rate of breathing. It was a horrible feeling. I thought I was about to die. The cumulative effect of the stress on my lungs from running so fast, and the anxiety I felt about not being able to breath resulted in a panic so severe I nearly lost consciousness. My breath returned in less than a minute, but it seemed like I had endured hours of a torture worse than being forced to watch <u>Pitch Perfect 2</u>.

As frightened as I was, I did not panic as I fought for breath that early morning. I imagined my lungs to be as strong as they were when I finished that ten-kilometer race. I pictured my lungs as being stronger and more resilient than the Coronavirus. I thought that the hard work of running so many races, completing so may marathons had provided me with a vast lung capacity, prodigious enough to see me through to the end of this race.

To reduce any anxiety that might work contrary to my resoluteness while I forced each breath, I turned on my television. I found a station that was playing the James Cagney film Footlight Parade. It was a favorite of mine; I was amazed by Cagney's irrepressible optimism and singing and dancing talents. By the time he performed "Shanghai Lil" I noticed that I was no longer conscious of or worried about my breathing; it had returned to its normal pattern.

At the end of "Shanghai Lil" Busby Berkeley added an appreciative nod of recognition to FDR for his leadership during a time of world crisis. At that moment I was reminded that no one, apart from Fox News employees and White House Cabinet members, would orchestrate a similar salute to our President for his handling of the Coronavirus crisis.

The next step in my struggle to breathe freely was to see if a reclined position with the television off would facilitate normal breathing. I struggled with a fair degree of trepidation about a move which I considered extreme.

Once I was back in bed, I closed my eyes and thought about other Cagney movies like Yankee Doodle Dandy. If that film were remade in our current environment, "Over There" would surely become "Over Here." The George M. Cohan character might not be thanking the President for a Congressional Gold Medal because, unlike Franklin Delano Roosevelt, our President might decide that he himself was a more proper recipient That was my last conscious thought before I fell asleep. My shortness of breath was gone three hours after it had raised its ugly head.

When I got myself out of bed at 1 p.m. that afternoon I decided to see if what I had experienced that morning had been reported as a typical COVID-19 symptom in any literature. I drew a blank and concluded that it was an event that led patients to require either a supplemental oxygen source or a ventilator. While I prepared the drink that I had begun to refer to as my Ninja Nuke, I prayed that my breathing episode had been a one and off encounter.

Sonia leapt onto my granite countertop to find the source of the strange noise she was hearing. She watched as I debated which of the Ninja's three labor-saving blending options I should use. There was a Smoothie button, a Ninja-Blend button, and a Ninja-Ultra-Blend button. When I pressed the Smoothie button she bolted and ran to hide under my green leather sofa, safe from the disturbingly sudden and loud, ugly noise generated by the Ninja. Her head was visible sticking out of the front of the sofa between her two gray and white paws.

I approached her slowly, and my heart went out to her when I looked down and saw bubbles of moisture emerging from the tip of her nose. My poor cat had no understanding that she had FIP and that her breathing would always be labored. It was a thought that shook me to the core of my being, one that sent my consciousness reeling. I knew I was facing a serious threat to my life and I was scared. How much scarier it must be, I thought, *not* to know one's life was threatened, and to experience only the painful symptoms of a disease. Like COVID-19 patients who did not know they were sick, Sonia was not aware that something bad was happening to her. I knew I was sick, and I knew I did not know the exact nature of the disease or what to do next. Sonia did not possess that first or second level of awareness. The thought caused me to cry in sympathy for her plight and for the struggle in which all COVID-19 patients were engaged.

Sonia viewed me not as a human but as a Very Big Cat. Once she bonded with me, I became her mother figure. She could trust me to protect her from the dangers of an unpredictable world. She felt a relaxed affection which resulted from her assuredness that I would never cause her any harm. She wandered freely around my home, confident that it was her fortress, one which would keep what had happened to her when she was abandoned as a kitten from happening again. I wished I could communicate to her that I was doing my best to keep her alive, and that was why I was giving her a disagreeable decongestant. It was as though a more sentient being from another galaxy or dimension observed those of us suffering from COVID-19 and thought, "Those poor things, they don't know how to solve this rudimentary biological problem."

How horrible it must also be, I thought, if, like Sonia, I was not to be able to cough or expectorate. I would be in trouble if I could not cough to clear out some Coronavirus gunk from my lungs. From that moment on, I viewed coughing as part of a cure, not as the curse I had previously regarded it to be.

To coax her from her point of retreat, I sat next to her, made eye contact, and blinked at her. She blinked back and climbed into my lap. I brushed her with one of the spikey cat brushes I keep in various spots around my home. I had discovered that gently brushing the sides of her head below her eyes and behind her chin stimulated a sneeze response. After a minute of this grooming she sneezed repeatedly, and each time she did, I positively reinforced each sneeze with a falsetto echoing of "Yea! Good kitty!" This never failed to activate her "more sneezing" button, and in less than sixty seconds she had gotten rid of the liquid that had caused her nose to run. I gave her some Viralys and offered her some green tea, which she declined to sample.

This event reminded me that I needed to avoid over-reacting to problems. Although it felt like everything in my body had gone haywire, being anxious or feeling desperate about my or her condition would increase the strength and frequency of our symptoms. Achieving a detached perspective, though, was easier said than done. I knew firsthand that every other illness I have experienced would fix itself with time or therapy. I had no such knowledge about COVID-19. I did not believe it would resolve itself with time, and there was no known therapy or vaccine in existence. It was therefore difficult not to let worst-case fears run rampant.

As I experienced this irresoluteness, I found that praying provided me with the restorative that I needed. I viewed the presence of God in my life to be as the Jesuit philosopher and scientist Pierre Teilhard de Chardin described in his second book, Hymn of the Universe. He wrote, "God is not remote from us. He is at the point of my pen, my pick, my paintbrush, my needle—and my heart and my thoughts." I wished that our President could demonstrate the compassion that is a natural outgrowth of faith, that he would recognize the truth of the philosopher's words that "We are not human beings having a spiritual experience. We are spiritual beings having a human experience." I wished that someday our President would allow spirituality to enter his life, but if wishes were horses, beggars would ride.

I wondered what lesson we must learn from having such a myopic man as President during the Coronavirus pandemic. Perhaps we should prohibit future Republican candidates from stealing elections. Perhaps we should demand a complete revamping of the Electoral College. While we are in corrective mode, maybe we should ask President Trump nicely to stop writing Dear John letters to Dr. Tedros Adhanom Ghebreyesus, Director General of the World Health Organization. Perhaps we can convince him to continue to fund an organization upon which most of the world depends, particularly so during a pandemic. I am afraid, though, that acquiescence to perform a humanitarian gesture would be borne from a sense of compassion which our President lacks.

Perhaps the too-little, too-late measures he took to address this pandemic will provide a lesson for the future. Perhaps it will gear us up for a later struggle with a more lethal Superflu, one which would be immediately fatal to ninety-nine percent of mankind, one that followed a progression to match the one Stephen King described in Chapter Fourteen of The Stand. In that novel, Colonel Deitz reported to his superiors, "We've got a disease that's got several well-defined stages...but some people may skip a stage. Some people may backtrack a stage. Some people may do both. Some people stay in one stage for a relatively long time and others zoom through all four as if they were in a rocket-sled...it scares me because nobody but a very smart doctor with all the facts is going to be able to diagnose anything but a common cold in the people who are out there carrying this... So they are going to stay home, drink fluids and get plenty of bedrest, and then they're going to die. Before they do, they're going to infect everyone who comes into the same room with them."[43]

I would dread being one of the persons "who comes into the same room with" President Trump. He would be the asymptomatic but contagious person in the room who chose not to wear a mask. Four and a half more years of learning lessons from President Trump's missteps would not be survivable, even if for the entire time we chose to "stay home, drink fluids and get plenty of bedrest." If I left home, I certainly would not visit Las Vegas based on what happened at the end of The Stand.

As difficult as it is for me to avoid feeling despondent in the Trump era, my wellbeing depended on my ability to maintain an overwhelming sense of optimism, and to retain a cheery outlook on my chances of recovering from a disease I was convinced I had contracted. I admit it is discouraging to watch our President conduct a "rally 'round the Space Force flag," for example, and listen to his "Super-Duper Missile" sabre rattling speeches without panicking.

But being a Gloomy Gus was no way to go through life. I attempted to focus on the positive. I was about to embark on an all-in, life-saving adventure, one which I should view with excitement and enthusiasm. I accepted the fact that the fight would pose severe physical and emotional challenges and I knew that there was no time like the present to begin. I had seen Simon Curtis' 2019 film <u>The Art of Racing in the Rain</u>, and I recalled Formula One driver Denny Swift (Milo Ventimiglia) saying, "No race was won on the first corner, but many were lost there." I decided April 3 would be my first corner.

Denny Swift's story was told from the point of view of his dog Enzo. Swift loved Enzo, and when he found Enzo whimpering near his door and not greeting him as he always did when Swift returned home, he knew that Enzo was approaching the end of his days on Earth. Enzo had often watched Denny racing toward a finish line. Denny knew that above all other treats, Enzo would most appreciate a ride with him on the racetrack. He gave Enzo that ride, and after a final lap around a Formula One track, Enzo asked for just one more time, one last lap, and Denny obliged.

When Sonia's final days approach, when she comes to the last of her nine lives, I will do for her the one thing I know she enjoys most. If she can no longer jump high enough, I will place her gently on my desk chair, and watch her as she stands on her back legs, clutches the top of the chair's back with her front paws, and peers out at the world over the top of the chair, with her pupils dilated in excitement. I would then rotate the chair, slowly at first, then ever more quickly, until the chair completed a rotation every three seconds. Her eyes would widen further, and with each spin, her head would turn to view the oncoming horizon from a renewed vantage point.

After I engaged her in her favorite play activity for an hour, I would let the chair slow to a stop. She would look at me at that point, and like Enzo, she would request a few last spins. I would of course oblige her, I would keep spinning the chair until she released her grasp of the chair's top, which signaled that she has had enough fun and was ready to jump off.

She would then climb into the open, lower drawer of my dresser, where she would snuggle in, on top of my socks and sweatshirts and pajamas, and begin to purr.

Like Enzo and Sonia asking for one more go-round, each night I prayed to God to please grant me one more spin, let me experience one more rotation of the Earth on its axis, and if it is in His Infinite Plan, perhaps one more sun cycle. It was a wish I knew I shared with all COVID-19 patients.

I do not know which sort of Coronavirus causes FIP in cats, but I suspected that the disease was not a natural occurrence. The species would have been decimated long ago if that had been the case. It is more likely that man had screwed with the environment in some foul way, and now cats suffered the consequences of our actions. President Trump's negligent and harmful misdeeds have more than sufficiently screwed with our chances of surviving the Coronavirus pandemic, and although I was often sickened by what I saw, it was neither helpful nor sustainable to exist in a constant state of anger and frustration. Those were the natural reactions when confronted by an Administration that prided itself on its record of nonexistent accomplishments and wallowing in the ignorance of its dangerously abhorrent complacency, but they would not help us survive when the rent came due.

Denny Swift also knew that if he could visualize the course, he could master it, because "When I'm in the race car, I'm the creator of my own destiny." Those words rang clear and true. I decided firmly and unequivocally that I would drive this car to the finish line, and I would win a race of one. I repeated Swift's mantra until I could see myself having completely recovered from COVID-19. I resolved to make my outlook on this matter positive, unchangeable, and adamantine.

Each time I turned on my television I was reminded that our chief politicians' intent was also ironclad. They used every opportunity to cash in on the presence of the Coronavirus in our society and created their own opportunities when none were present. The President and Vice President disregarded the record-setting number of positive test cases in June, July, and August 2020, all of which had resulted from states moving too quickly to re-open.

On June 24, Vice-President Pence was spurred to action by a President hoping to recover from the embarrassment of the low turnout for the Tulsa rally. Pence encouraged our Governors to identify with Jonah in the whale and accentuate the positive aspects of life in the Trump reign and eliminate the negative consequence of one hundred and fifty thousand American deaths caused by the pandemic, or rather, by the President's nightmarish and bungled efforts to control the spread of the pandemic. Neither man accepted plausible, alternate, safe scenarios for saving the nation; there was no Mister In-Between.

Although the number of positive cases and consequently, the number of hospitalizations and deaths from COVID-19 were setting record highs every day since Memorial Day, we were told by a head-in-the-sand Administration that everything was fine, that we should move along because there was nothing to see here. It was another poignant example of Executive misguidance, of an engineer sitting at the throttle of a run-away train with his eyes closed, while the conductor announced to all passengers, "Everything's under control, our speed is one hundred percent correct for this stretch of track." Like any strategy that substituted fiction for fact, that ignored inherent complexities, that denied the likelihood of dangerous and long-term consequences, our Administration's plan to re-open states was doomed from the onset.

Many of our largest corporations have turned similar blind eyes to the ongoing pandemic. Walmart is facing a wrongful death lawsuit for its mishandling of a COVID-19 outbreak in its Evergreen Park, Illinois store. Kroger ended its employee bonus program. McDonald's workers in Chicago sued the company for "failing to safeguard the health of staff and customers." Darden Restaurants, which owns Olive Garden and LongHorn Steakhouse brands, furloughed one hundred and fifty thousand of its minimum wage workers. The list was endless.

I lost the small sense of composure I was feeling one evening when I saw a Starbuck's television commercial which promoted its newest flavored beverage, which was a mango and dragonfruit drink. The image of dragonfruit slices dancing and swirling joyfully in an animated background bore a striking resemblance to the standard, magnified picture we have come to recognize as the Novel Coronavirus. I understood that many people of Chinese ancestry believe a dragon is a symbol of good luck coming their way, but I wondered why a keen-sighted executive of the firm had not objected, "Wait a minute. How are we supposed to sell a new product when the Coronavirus is one of its two main ingredients?" Apparently, our President was not alone in his misguided attempt to color our perception of what is real when he recently called COVID-19 the Kung Flu and the Invisible China Virus.

Nevertheless, no matter how many stupid actions I witnessed our President performing, I was determined not be discouraged. No matter how often he assaulted my sensibilities and attacked the foundations of freedom which protect me, I would not be deterred. My resolve to detach and stay on course would be tested when, contrary to all medical advice, President Trump ordered churches throughout our country to re-open. That action, and its implication that his *professed* commitment to spirituality required churches to open prematurely, demonstrated his penchant for one-step thinking.

I have always found the non-thinking part of his essence of ignorance to be unacceptably cloying. In this case my irritation was worsened by the knowledge that Mr. Trump's motivation was political, not spiritual. From April 3 onward, I would take note of these examples of Presidential equivocating. I would view with disdain his solecisms, his inactions, his dumb decisions, like hosting a three-thousand person, no-social-distancing-acceptable church rally in Phoenix on June 23, 2020.

Joe Strummer and Mick Jones expressed a relevant sentiment in their lyric, "London calling to the imitation zone/Forget it, brother, you can go it alone." I understood that when they sang "go it alone," they meant without an iota of spiritual, physical, or emotional assistance from Whitehall. I agreed. I would not expect any help from the current administration of our government, which lived and breathed an imitation zone defined by lies and denials.

Then again, perhaps President Trump could serve us as an opposite barometer. If he did not wear a mask, the rest of us should not venture outside without wearing a mask. When the three thousand people at his June 23 Phoenix church rally saw that the President, who was not wearing a mask, planned to address them in a setting too up close and personal for their safety or his, they should have run from their seats as though the

Dream City Megachurch was one of the Seven Gates of Hell. And yet, unbelievably, acting contrary to the best advice of scientific community, they remained seated, oblivious to the danger the setting represented and shouted and cheered for the demagogue at the pulpit. Any sane individual would not sit down too close to a rattlesnake nest and wait to see what happened when they poked the sidewinders with a stick, unless they were convinced by the ophidians that they were not in mortal danger.

I will never understand why those three thousand festivalgoers did not recognize the importance of physical distancing. Birds, rabbits, squirrels, feral cats, deer, and the occasional coyote all have IQ's at least equal to those of the people attending the Phoenix rally. If wild animals can understand that it is not safe for them to be too close to a human, then why couldn't those people manifest a commensurate level of the instinct for self-preservation? The only explanation I can propose is that a lemming gene exists in the DNA of Trump supporters.

Starting April 3, no matter how terrible I felt, I vowed there would be no skipping meals, no skipping of Nutri Nukes, vitamins, minerals, liquids, exercises, or anything else that might help battle COVID-19. I decided that each morning I would wait a few hours before doing thirty-five sit ups, because I wanted to avoid jostling the liquids that were already sloshing around in my stomach.

I was glad to have survived the night, and I was excited and anticipatory because I was already three-days into the three-to-five-day waiting period for hearing the results of my March 31 test. At any moment my phone could ring and I could be talking to I hope a human from Test Results who very conceivably would tell me I was not infected, thank you very much for waiting in your car all morning and consuming a test that could have been better spent on a person who was actually sick. Click. If that was the case, I would not have to drink another Ninja Nuke or do another set of sit-ups.

I looked at my Nutri Ninja. Its buttons and display board seemed to sneer at me, defying me to attempt to make another Nuke. Sonia yawned. I could tell that the towering and ominous presence of the Nutri Ninja did not bother her. She was planning the rest of her busy day and evening, contemplating when to visit the litterbox; when to take her next nap; when to investigate the goings-on of the robins eating the birdseed I had distributed on my balcony's concrete floor on the other side of a glass door which was never seemed to be open long enough for her to venture outside; when to give me her "It's Dinnertime!" meow; when to stare at something I could not see near the ceiling; and when to run as fast as felinely possible into my study in the adjacent room for a reason unquantifiable by me but very clear to her.

Social distancing measures were extended by Presidential announcement until the end of April. I had left home once to go shopping. I had worn one of the surgical masks in my toolbox, which I had purchased a month ago when I had planned to sand and re-varnish my kitchen cabinetry. I had tried to keep my distance from mask-less shoppers who invaded my personal space, the people who seemed determine to meet me head on in every aisle of every store, asking me to grab a can of lima beans or a box of mac and cheese from a top shelf that they could not reach, jockeying for a position closer to the cash register in the middle of a long checkout line in which I waited.

These Chicagoland shopping behaviors were beginning to feel off-kilter in early April. When the importance of physical distancing was more widely understood, most of us adapted to the new environment. Thanks to the urging of our Governor, we wore masks, we stayed home, and we prayed we would not become ill. By mid-May, that landscape began to change. Those individuals who followed social distancing measures were ostracized by those who did not. Wearing a mask and keeping six feet apart were viewed as tired, unnecessary, and pointless gestures. A formidable backlash had been spawned throughout the nation thanks to the abominable example our miscreant President had set.

By Memorial Day, our country had largely retreated to a position far worse than where we were when the pandemic first infiltrated our country. President Trump taunted Americans who practiced social distancing, and his supporters expressed their belligerence by refusing to follow any and every form of mitigation. Those of us who grasped the magnitude of the COVID-19 problem wore masks and stayed home. We understood that safety was more important than getting a suntan on Daytona Beach, but we were quickly becoming members of an endangered minority. An "Emperor Has No Mask" mentality prevailed, with millions of Americans believing that if the President of the United States thinks it is safe not to wear a mask, then it must be so.

By the end of May, most states yielded to the pressures exerted by President Trump. Though they failed to meet the minimum federal criteria suggested by the CDC for re-opening, they moved themselves into Phase One and beyond. The imperative expressed in "London Calling" became more relevant. Sooner or later, governors would realize that to survive COVID-19, they would need to form alliances with each other for two reasons: President Trump would not help them, and the Coronavirus did not respect state borders.

Interstate inconsistencies were made more difficult to resolve because lines of authority within the state, from city to city, from county to county, from the governor's office to cities and counties were muddled. Atlanta Mayor Keisha Lance Bottoms for example ordered a mask ordinance in her city; Georgia Governor Brian Kemp countermanded her order and forbid her to institute that life-saving policy. Iowa Governor Kim Reynolds declared that Iowa City Mayor Bruce Teague did not have the authority to issue a mask ordinance.

Like hundreds of other political skirmishes, this foray into insanity could have been avoided if a national face covering ordinance had been enacted. With our Lord Cardigan to blame for our Light Brigade charge to re-open the country, there was no chance in hell of such an ordinance finding a place on the drawing board.

It occurred to me that I should use each distressing piece of news about more bureaucratic foul-ups as a motivator. Every time I heard our President play fast and loose with the facts, I would add another component to my proactive struggle to feel better. For example, if I heard that the Dow was up because the Fed was buying junk bonds, I would say a rosary. When unemployment figures rose to forty million claims, I would drink an extra glass of grapefruit juice. If Avis followed Hertz Car Rentals in filing for bankruptcy, I would do ten extra sit ups.

When I learned that air travel from Brazil was banned and that the corpses piling up in Rio De Janeiro's barrios rivaled the heights of stacks of bodies in the streets of Quito, Ecuador, I would perform an extra five minutes of breathing exercises, covering my mouth with the warm, damp washcloth I had been using to add moisture to my lungs. Because I did not want to alarm my neighbors, that washcloth also served me well in stifling any screams of frustration that political announcements might elicit from me.

Upon seeing that number of COVID-19-infected workers in our country's meat processing facilities had risen to eighteen thousand, I decided not to order for delivery the Number Three Chick-Fil-A dinner. Instead I would call my local Lou Malnati's and would ask the friendly order-taker to please have a large, butter-crust, deep dish, cheese pizza delivered to my door in an hour. I would happily perform this action, knowing that I was making lemonade of the lemons President Trump threw at me. This would be my Clash remediation strategy, and it would lessen my anger over countless examples of Presidential ineptitude. It would reduce my level of frustration over the endless daily barrage of Coronavirus mis-dealings and lies that came my way. It would reduce the hopeless, tired anxiety I felt every time I saw the President on television—and I did not even watch <u>Fox News</u>.

I needed to set upper limits for these added-value categories. For example, two hundred sit-ups a day would be a maximum number to achieve; more than two glasses of grapefruit juice would probably upset my stomach; one or two rosaries a day would suffice; and I should probably limit pizza consumption to one large Lou's per week. I recognized that with the mounting number of political and sociological missteps taken by the President, my ability to respond in kind would be as taxed as an ICU unit in Harris County, Texas.

I would need to prorate my actions on a ten per one basis. For every ten reports of water park parties held in places like Lake of the Ozarks, Missouri, I would perform only one of the above actions. I could add more categories of response as needed. No single plan is perfect when fighting COVID-19, but I was confident mine would work well enough for me. I took each depressing news report quite seriously, because now was not the time for glibness or sarcasm.

It broke my heart to learn that the absence of any federal testing plan had led to an extraordinarily high infection and death rate in the Navajo

Nation, and that four out of every ten residents of nursing homes in the United States had died from COVID-19. My remediation plan was my defense mechanism for coping with the mind-numbingly, overwhelmingly dissociative statements and decisions made by our indolent and feckless President.

I realized that, from the outside, it might appear as though I was playing irrational and needless mind games, but I propose that it is not easy to find an equilibrium when suffering from COVID-19. My day had become as full as Sonia's. I prepped my dinner before doing my sit-ups. The deep breathing exercises I performed every other hour reduced my coughing for a while, and cough drops allowed me to sit for longer periods of time, but menthol does not mesh well with olive oil and parmesan, and my few functioning taste buds rejected the idea. Because the adrenalin produced from exercising lessened my appetite, I adjusted my schedule and did not exercise too soon before a meal.

I could not wait too long afterwards, however, because my breathing exercises quickly lost their effectiveness and I would end up battling a coughing fit while staring at a plateful of pasta going cold. I also had to contend with the lump of pills that I swallowed before eating. Although there was no discernible taste when swallowed quickly with grapefruit juice, I felt like they were taking up a good amount of stomach space, floating around down there until they dissolved. It was better to wait a few minutes before rushing too abruptly into a heavy meal, but every bottle of fat-soluble pills in my cabinet had a label which read, "take with food."

Sitting in my recliner exacerbated the urge to cough, but I could not eat while laying on my back. I watched the day's live Coronavirus Task Force briefings while eating dinner, but it was difficult to watch Donald Trump's footlight parade without ruining what little appetite of mine had remained.

I was confident that in a day or two I would find an ideal solution to this curious puzzle of conflicting interactions. I had not guessed that eating would become so complicated when COVID-19 factored itself into the equation. No wonder none of the Wuhan residents cared whether they got a bowl of rice at dinnertime or not. Since I found it unsettling to watch Task Force briefing on my fifty-inch, curved QLED Samsung monitor while I sat in my fancy leather recliner in my warm living room, twirling forkfuls of pasta and eating unenthusiastically with Sonia in my lap, I could not imagine how badly the innocent victims living in Wuhan City must have felt sitting alone in their plastic chairs in a cold, nameless warehouse hallway, without comfort or console, their minds filled with fear of the unknown, their bodies aching for a release from a type of pain they had never heretofore experienced, from which there was no escape. They must have felt the same despair our nursing home residents experienced when they watched one out of every two of their sick friends leave in an ambulance and never return, while they themselves wondered if the next day the piper would call them to their final resting place. I promised myself I would not go gently or otherwise into the Coronavirus night.

My natural inclination was to lay down after eating, so that I would feel less like coughing, but I had heard that doing so was bad for the heart and acted as an acid reflux contributor, so I resorted to lemon cough drops while reading for an hour. I never read in bed, because that practice inculcated a bad habit of reading to go to sleep. Once that action was in play, reading would become a cause for drowsiness while sitting.

Television however was a perfect somnolent. I could not watch very many political news shows or listen to late night commentators because the information was too stimulating. I would change channels after Anderson Cooper's show on <u>CNN</u> and Rachel Maddow's on <u>MSNBC</u> ended, and I would search for something amusingly enervated and sufficiently vapid to watch until I fell asleep. A show like <u>Storage Wars</u> or a movie like <u>The Towering Inferno</u> served that purpose quite well.

One night I was lucky to catch a commercial-free broadcast of the demented 1986 Wolfgang Peterson film <u>Poseidon</u>. I was glad the director had returned to the familiar underwater territory which was the setting he last explored in 1981 when he directed the film <u>Das Boot</u>. Seeing normal activity on a cruise ship before it was hit by a rogue wave was lurid in its appeal. If the image of social interaction on a cruise ship was appealing, then contemplating taking an actual cruise was visceral in its level of excitement. When I watched Richard Widmark ride a crowded New York subway train in the 1953 Sam Fuller film <u>Pick Up on South Street</u> I yearned to return to the days of steerage transport on Chicago's Blue Line.

I was not surprised by Carnival Cruise Lines' announcement that its ships would sail again in September. If that timeline is met, cruising in the era of Coronavirus will not resemble cruising as we had come to know it for the past four decades. The example of seven hundred positive cases of COVID-19 on the Diamond Princess demonstrated that cruising fell in the highest category of risk for likely transmission of the Coronavirus. A cruise ship vacation qualified as a "Super Spreader," as defined by Dr. Birx, because a great amount of activity would take place indoors in a crowded space. Outdoor activity would also be crowded, and there would be a fair amount of shouting, which was a mode of transmission that the Coronavirus found to be eminently viable. Whether indoors or outdoors, activities would take place over a long period of time. Vacationers would share food and drinks.

It is difficult to imagine a scenario worse than taking a cruise if anyone wished to remain COVID-19 free. The Coronavirus agenda did *not* include dying of its own accord when so many willing subjects offered themselves as infectees whenever they rolled the dice at the craps table or used the same ladle to fill their plates with scalloped potatoes and sauerkraut at the midnight buffet. The Coronavirus would look at the printed itinerary of next day activities that every guest received under their door each night and would think gleefully, "Wow, looks like we will have a record-setting day at Atlantis on Paradise Island tomorrow!"

That was a future worry. I had a more immediate concern, and it involved my cat. An hour after her April 2 dose of decongestant, the edges of Sonia's ears had turned crimson. I withheld giving her any decongestant on April 3. I was treading a narrow path with her. Decongestants helped her clear her lungs, but it sometimes caused a mild allergic reaction. Her red tipped ears were a sign for me to back off for a day or two until her ears returned to their normal, dark gray color. Then I would only give her one-half a milliliter and see if that caused a reaction. I had a nagging feeling that there was a lesson to be learned here, but because I could not define its meaning or place it in context, the fuller thought remained dormant.

I could continue with her Viralys treatments because they had never caused a similar reaction after I gave her a fingertip-full of that stuff. I would say that my motivation to have her survive FIP was equal to my own drive to recover from my troublesome symptoms. To look at the situation from another angle, I was never a sportsman. I have never gone hunting and I had fished only twice, from a rowboat on a Wisconsin lake with my father and grandfather. I had philosophical and practical reasons for not hunting. I wanted all creatures to enjoy as much of a full-term life as possible. The fact that I was afraid of guns, knives, bows and arrows, and other implements of destruction would have limited my ability to hunt had I been morally and ethically inclined to do so. I also did not fare well with heights and I was not on friendly terms with most insects. Oddly enough, there was little chance of me dying from a gunshot wound or a stabbing or falling from the ninety-fifth floor of the Hancock Building in the immediate future, but those horrible possibilities were palm-sweating scary. COVID-19 on the other hand could very capably deliver me to that same fate and I was determined not to let that likelihood frighten me.

I certainly wanted Sonia to live a safe, full, and pleasant life. I had rescued her as a kitten from underneath a wood-framed home where she had been abandoned by a negligent owner who moved away in the dead of night. I remember that day quite vividly because three Chicago police cars and a tactical unit arrived the next day to search the premises for its contents and its nowhere to be found owner. Rumor had it that an illegal drug operation had precipitated the raid.

I carried Sonia home and inspected her. She had fleas. I removed the ones I could spot in her short hair and ears and I bathed her in my bathroom sink. To this day, when she is frightened by thunder, she returns to that sink. What I learned from her method of seeking sanctuary was that we all need a place to retreat when overwhelmed by life. Some people find refuge in a bottle. Some find it in a hefty meatball sandwich. My place was figurative, and I never failed to find it whenever I talked to God.

After prayers that night I decided to be happy with the progress I had made in the past ten hours. April 3 had provided me with a daily model for the weeks, perhaps months to come. I would sleep as late as I could each day, which would allow my immune system to repair itself from whatever tricks the Coronavirus had played on it that day. I would take my temperature and swallow an Excedrin Extra or two if my headache warranted it. I would exercise, shave and shower, and take vitamins with my Ninja Nuke, with green tea as a chaser. When I added oatmeal and raisins to my ersatz breakfast menu, I was no longer able to endorse lunch as a formal concept. My afternoon was free to nap, search online for new Coronavirus information, and contemplate which variety of pasta and vegetables would be suitable for dinner.

For recreation I would spend about two hours a day amusing Sonia with various parlor tricks. She responded with wide-eyed interest every time I made a scratching noise with my fingertips on an object outside of her field of vision. It was fun to watch how her telescopic ears could fix precisely on the location of a hidden noise ten feet from her. She would then run and pounce on where my finger had been, thinking that she was helping me locate the mysterious animal that had invaded our home and was creating such an audible disturbance. Hers was a cautionary tale, warning me not to mistake cause for effect when battling COVID-19.

She had cultivated a nice habit of crawling onto my shoulder when I sat at my desk and worked. Despite her close proximity to my ear I could not hear her purr because her breathing was too wheezy, but I could tell she was very happy in that position while I tried in a cramped way to type and use my mouse without moving my shoulders. I did not want to upset the precarious applecart upon which she was perched. Most of the time I stopped what I was doing and allowed her to sit on my chest and shoulder for as long as she wanted to remain there. I refuse to live with regrets, and I knew that someday I would regret not having allowed her to enjoy more time with me in a pose that made her happy.

In the past Sonia would run and hide whenever I sat on the edge of my bed and practiced on one of two guitars. For a while I thought it was her way of commenting on the quality of my playing. At first, she had run for cover whenever I reached to remove either my Les Paul Traditional Electric or my Martin acoustic guitar from its stand. Somewhere along the line she decided she could tolerate the Martin, but she shied away from my blood orange flamed Les Paul, even if it was unplugged. I concluded it was the songs I played on the Martin, not the guitar that appealed to her body and soul. She seemed to prefer Bob Dylan songs, and one of her favorites was called "Billy." Whenever she heard its supple rhymes, its predictably reassuring chord pattern of G, C major, and D, its "some sweet senorita" sibilance, she would lick her paws, wipe her face, and lie patiently on her back with legs akimbo, where she would remain until I finished the last line, "Billy you're so far away from home." I would reward her attentiveness by rubbing her stomach. Over the years she had become a good listener and a faithful fan.

She made it clear to me that she disliked hearing the electric intro solo to "Sweet Child O' Mine," but she would sit motionless and stare transfixed whenever she saw the sixty-second spot for Trulicity on television. She ran like hell to escape any commercial advertisement for Geico. I concluded that Trulicity's calm visuals appealed to her, but its big selling point was the way the word "Trulicity" sounded. The half-rhyme was close enough to "kitty" to be pleasing to her ear, as was the "Billy" melody. Clearly the image of an animated gecko and the jarring dissonance of it voice were as scary for her as my Les Paul riffs, and probably had frightened her as much as the movies Vertical Limit, Daylight, The Deadly Bees, and Arachnophobia had scared the hell out of me. I decided to play my Les Paul on my balcony with the glass door shut, to her relief and to the unfettered annoyance of my neighbors.

After I retrieved the mail each afternoon and decided which pieces needed baking or burning, I spent some time reading for fun. There was a book of poetry called Expresslanes Through the Inevitable City that interested me; I liked the way the poems, written as though they were blues songs, celebrated Chicago's Chess Records heritage. I spent an hour each day reading JFK and the Unspeakable: Why He Died and Why It Matters by historian and Catholic theologian James W. Douglass. I was halfway through his massive work and I agreed with Oliver Stone's assessment that it was "the best account I have read of this tragedy and its significance." I was amazed by how eloquently Douglass illustrated Kennedy's intelligence, integrity, compassion, and moral authority. I wished our current President possessed one of those four qualities.

I would have preferred to read for more than an hour, but after sixty minutes my arms ached, my levee-breaking headache returned, and my vision became blurry. I used to be able to read for ten hours in a row, but those days, like my marathon-running days, were probably long gone. I hoped that like Wolfgang Peterson I could return to those familiar territories at some point in my future, but until then I would take baby steps, like the ones that Ted Arroway (David Morse) told his daughter Ellie (Jodie Foster) to take when encountering foreign landscapes in Robert Zemeckis' 1997 film Contact.

I was not working for a living, but then again, neither was I experiencing the life of Riley. I was enjoying the advantages of an early retirement with none of its benefits. I had been enrolled in Medicare Parts A, B, D, and G for three years and the system had worked well; I did not have very many medical bills to pay outside of my premiums. The fact that I was not working and consequently not receiving any paychecks did not bother me as much as it might have if I did not have COVID-19 symptoms to manage. Financial concerns seemed far removed from my horizon. I had saved enough money to support a modest lifestyle, and any problem that I encountered that could be fixed with money was not a problem. I knew that I would never be able to buy an Aston Martin DBS V12 which was my dream car ever since I saw Daniel Craig as James Bond drive it in <u>Casino Royale</u>. If I could afford such wonderful piece of automotive craftsmanship, my lifestyle would no longer be considered modest.

Had I owned the Aston Martin I could not have driven it anywhere, like Joe Walsh lamented about his Maserati in "Life's Been Good." My afternoon schedule was full and would not yield to hedonistic bends. Before prepping my dinner, I had laundry to do, consisting of towels, sheets, pillowcases, washcloths, t-shirts, sweatpants, and pajamas. Then I would either spray with a disinfectant or wipe down with Isopropyl any surfaces I had touched, especially my keyboard and tv remote. The rumor was that the Coronavirus lived longer on nonporous surfaces.

I used my Monster Screenclean spray on the screen of my laptop; when I coughed unexpectedly, I would invariably contaminate my laptop screen, making it unsanitary and harder to read. Once I was through with dinner, after the plates and utensils were stacked in my dishwasher, I would wipe down all kitchen surfaces while I decided which series of dessert items was most appealing. I would routinely give Sonia her fourth meal of the day before I verified that all doors were locked. I would then wash my hands and face, turn off the lights, and enjoy a few cookies and a candy bar or two while channel surfing between <u>CNN</u> and <u>MSNBC</u>. I would have my notebook and pen ready in case I was struck with a brainstorm in the middle of the night. I would jot down in a semi-conscious manner an idea that seemed to be brilliant at the time; most of those notations were illegible in the morning.

This was the pattern I would follow until I was either cured or hospitalized. As closely as I could figure, there remained two immediate variables: how I would feel the next day, and what dreams I might experience. I could monitor each of the two, but I could not predict the course that either would take. I would be happy if my temperature stayed below one hundred and one and if my blood pressure remained under one hundred and thirty over ninety. Coughing was a constant.

Some nights my dreams were as scattered and wild as any of Hunter Thompson's ether-induced hallucinations, filled with phantoms and chimera. Those types of dreams were not troublesome. Thirty-some years ago I had experimented with LSD and mescaline and I knew that those trips were ephemeral and posed no threat or greater significance. With a simple act of will, I could transform any unsettling, drug-induced specter into a series of wondrous imagery, scenarios where barren, gray fields would give way to beautiful and comforting terrains. Pooneil Corners, for example, would become verdant forests "where the trees have leaves of prisms that break the light into colors that no one knows the names of."[44] My current hallucinatory dreams like those trips were easily understandable, and posed no threat to my emotional or psychological health. Similarly, though I could not control the content of those dreams, I was not frightened by their weirdness.

The dreams that puzzled me were the ones I have previously mentioned, populated by presences that some people might call spirits of the dead trying to communicate with me. Such a reading was freakishly bothersome to me. However, if I approached the topic as any competent symbologist would, my task was clearer and less disturbing. What if the dream I was experiencing was interpretive, not prophetic in nature? What if my subconscious had neatly personalized the concept of death for me because the enormity of the scale of COVID-19 deaths in our country defied comprehension? I was happier proceeding from that more encouraging ontological perspective. There were no bad dreams, only ones with meanings I failed to recognize for a while.

To collect enough dream data, first thing every morning I recorded what I could remember of each dream, and I would review perhaps a week's worth of dreams at some later date. Confident in the efficacy of that solution, I took my aspirin, my Vitamin C, and my statin, and dozed off while watching the amusing byplay between Pierce Brosnan and Rene Russo on a Martinique beach in The Thomas Crown Affair. The last thing I remember that night was noticing that Brosnan drove a 1967 Mustang in that film, which was a wonderful piece of Shelby engineering but was not nearly as cool as the Vanquish model of the Aston Martin that Brosnan drove in Die Another Day, which was still a poor relation to Daniel Craig's DBS.

I wish I had dreamt about classic cars that night. Instead of finding myself strapped in for a test drive on a new silver Bentley Continental GT with a maroon interior, I saw myself sitting and waiting for an Amazon delivery of ink cartridges for my printer. Without those cartridges I could not complete a project which seemed significant at the time. When I awoke at 10 a.m. I did not remember any of the project specifics, but the meaning of the dream about waiting was clear. It was past time for me to receive a phone call from the Illinois Department of Public Health.

I found my Community Based Testing Site leaflet in a bedside stack of important papers. It had gotten shuffled between my Cubs schedule and an expired Costco ad paper featuring a deal on a new set of Michelin tires. I had intended to buy four of the Pilot Sport A/S +3s before it snowed on December 30, but I decided that I should get a haircut instead. Besides, if I limited my winter driving and waited until April to go to Costco, after the snow was gone, I would not have to spend five hundred dollars that day. Michelin tires would surely be on sale by then. In my worst-case scenario, I would buy a set of tires at on sale during the Memorial Day weekend. Due to a series of obvious and unfortunate events, tire-buying in April and May was postponed.

I had reached the far end of the three-to five-day window within which I should have received test results. I had no choice but to call the IDPH on April 4. I had a suspicion, more of an educated guess that making the call would be a lengthy endeavor, so after dialing and fighting my way through eight different menus and options, I was not surprised when a robot voice informed me that I should wait for the next representative because my call was important.

The call was quite important to me, but I could not gauge its relative importance to the ID of PH, since my projected wait time was between ninety and one hundred and twenty minutes. I could not complain; I knew they were busy. But it would have been nice if a public health department had an emergency plan to gear up staff in case a public health emergency like a pandemic occurred on its watch, causing sixty thousand people to call the Department seeking public health advice. It seemed that this simple "if... then" equation had escaped notice by public health officials in Springfield who no doubt had plenty of advice to give, but not enough staff to spread the word. It reminded me of how there were many available lifeboats in Poseidon, but there were no hands-on-deck to launch them once they were filled with terrified customers.

I kept my phone close by and on speaker mode, and I set out to accomplish my morning routine. The hours passed quickly as I played with Sonia. While watching the 2 p.m. news, I debated the pros and cons of hanging up. If I hung up, I would spend another day in test result limbo. If I stayed on the line, what were my chances of talking to anyone before business hours ended? Maybe there was an algorithm in place that identified the number from which I was calling IDPH, and then that number was cross-checked against the phone number that I gave to officials on my yellow post-it note at the Community Testing Site. If someone calling had only waited four days, for example, that call would go to the back burner.

It seemed to be farfetched concept, but it was possible. I plugged in my phone to recharge after three and a half more hours had passed; at the four-hour additional mark I gave up. If they wanted to test patience and resolve, I would play. In the unlikely event that an automatic, time-based screening process was in place, one which would limit calls being answered to the ones furthest outside the expected call-back time, I would give the Illinois Department of Public Health another few days. I hoped that for some indeterminable reason, whether it was algorithmic or serendipitous in nature, my next wait time would be less lengthy.

On the bright side, I had gleaned four important bits of information from my aborted attempt to speak with a representative. First, IDPH did not utilize the same auto-disconnect function favored by many bureaucracies that are too busy to talk to me. Second, eventually I would talk to a human because "the next available representative" could not be a computer. Third, IDPH needed to upgrade its on-hold music. Fourth, being on hold for six hours or more could push a persistent, mild headache from tolerable to eight-point-three Richter scale magnitude unless I reminded myself from time to time that I must not take IDPH's cold-shoulder personally.

The next three days were an exercise in discipline. I followed my routine, but I did not notice an improvement in my health. I had to admit that, objectively speaking, I felt worse each day. I did not blame the decline on any of my actions or lack of actions. I blamed it on the virulence of the Coronavirus.

I anxiously awaited news of my test results. I had been giving Sonia the lower dose of decongestant as planned, and her ears had returned to a grayer shade of pale. Clearly the size of the dose had an impact on her health. I wished I could lessen my symptoms so quickly.

One afternoon I was practicing guitar, playing some Beatles songs. I preferred to play along with ones that John sang, and that day I had been working on "Polythene Pam" from Abbey Road. I came to a dead standstill when the significance of the first two lines of the second stanza struck me. John sang, "Get a dose of her in jackboots and kilt/She's killer-diller when she's dressed to the hilt." Could the Coronavirus be my Polythene Pam? Would the virus be "killer-diller" for me only if it had been dressed to the hilt? Perhaps the dose of Coronavirus I received from The Sneeze was not of the size or comportment necessary to kill me.

I looked online and found that indeed the size of the dose, along with the age, the demographic, and general health of the victim *did* influence the severity of the illness and the victim's chance of recovery. Consequently, a positive test might not equal a death sentence for me. Maybe my Pam was topless and not dressed to the hilt. I found that to be an interesting and encouraging image, and I never tired of playing that song each day for the next seven weeks. Sonia grew tired of it, but I did not.

It was possible that I was completely wrong by thinking reductively about the size of the dose that I had received. Even if it turned out that my dose was of lethal scale, I was happy to discover a new way of looking at my problem. Prior to reducing Sonia's med and prior to playing that song I did not understand that the size of the dose affected the extremity of the cytokine storm. When I next talked to an Illinois Department of Public Health official, I would ask that person if they had any stats correlating dose sizes with Illinois deaths from COVID-19. Every day on the news a scientist or doctor would say that they are learning more and more about the nature of the Coronavirus. Surely someone at IDPH would have been watching the evening news and if so, he or she could share more specific information with me.

On April 7 I decided I had waited long enough. Each day the only message on my phone was a notice to update my Google Play services. Apparently my "drive won't run unless I updated" those services. The message struck me as odd because I use my old Escape android to make calls or respond to texts. I do not know how to go online with it. I had no idea what Google Play services were or why I had been selected to receive that message. It was another example of twenty-first century breakdown, similar to "caller unknown" voicemails handing me some malarkey about refinancing my home, or "urgent" emails from Holly Fiegerman telling me in the middle of February that "This portable air conditioner is HALF OFF today!"

I dialed the IDPH number, 800-889-3931, and selected option five. One minute later I was listening to those same dreadful songs on hold. One was Lawrence Welk's "Calcutta," which segued inexplicably into an elevator bossa nova. I recognized the Welk ditty from years of playing accordion when I was a twelve to fifteen- year-old boy. I wanted to play guitar, but that was not the instrument that a child in a Polish and Italian extended family was expected to master. In between IDPH songs, a human but not a live voice encouraged callers to visit dph.sick@illinois.gov. Since I had nothing better to do, I visited that website, though I wondered what positive outcome could be reasonably expected when going to a site that had the word "sick" as part of its address. I need not have worried, because, just like the www.cornonavirus .gov website, there was no new information on the IDPH site, no option for a live chat, no way to email them an inquiry. The earnest-sounding suggestion was an example of more electronic, Google Play nonsense.

As luck would have it, after thirty short minutes I heard a voice talking to someone in the background about chocolate sprinkled doughnuts before a woman addressed me with a "yes?" It was not as enthusiastic or polite of an opening gambit as I would have expected, but I welcomed it whole-heartedly. I quickly explained that I had been tested at the Community Based

Testing Site on Irving Park Road in Chicago on March 31, and I had not yet received a call about the results.

I asked if she could provide me with that information, because it had been eight days a week since I was tested and I was so tired, tired of waiting, tired of waiting for you. I was told in a clipped tone that due to the high number of tests that were given, results would not be forthcoming until ten to fourteen days. I found myself wishing I were talking to a robot when before hanging up, she said, "We will call people who were tested when we have results." The line was disconnected by her while I was saying "But I have a few questions..." One of my questions would have been, "How could the number of tests given be so unexpectedly high when you knew there were only two hundred and fifty tests allowed per day?" It was probably fortunate that our call ended before I could make that the rudimentary observation, because she might have taken the matter personally and might have branded me as a troublemaker. My name would be placed at the top of the list of people who would never receive another call from Test Results.

Fortune smiled on me two days later, when at 1040 a.m. on April 9 my phone rang. The caller I.D. told me that "Test Results" was on the line. My date with destiny had arrived.

Chapter Five

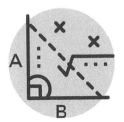

Results

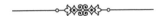

T he ten days I spent waiting for my call from IDPH were difficult ones. I was aware that a significant disparity in waiting time existed between the haves—the President and his staff—and the have nots— everyone else in the country. We did not have the luxury of being tested each day, with results disseminated ten minutes after a test was administered. Nor did we enjoy a test format easier to endure than the nasal swab which was de rigueur for Community Based Test Sites in March and April 2020. The White House used the Abbott ID Now protocol which President Trump called "highly accurate" but in fact misdiagnosed forty-eight percent of the samples taken.

Those of us who were not employed at 1600 Pennsylvania Avenue NW could be sick for a long while before realizing we might have COVID-19. Once determining that there was a possibility that we were so infected, we struggled to find a place where we would be accepted for testing. If we had not given up by that time and had located a possible test venue, we would wait in lines longer than the one I had encountered. At the end of June in Phoenix, for example, the line of applicants extended for a mile. Hundreds of people stood in line or sat on lawn chairs for thirteen hours, baking in the sun as they waited for an opportunity to be tested in Maricopa County. I suspected that some local political crony had acceded to the President's Tulsa rally request to "slow the testing down please," because testing could not possibly be going slower than the standstill represented by the Phoenix line. Health care providers at that site were powerless to meet the overwhelming demand for testing. They worked as hard as humanly possible to test everyone who had waited in line.

After being tested in March, we waited anywhere from five to fourteen days before receiving our result. I would guess that communication of said result went as well for me as it did for everyone who had spent hours, perhaps days in line at the Jackie Joyner Kersee Center in East St. Louis, Missouri, at 1412 Fairmount Avenue in Philadelphia, Pennsylvania, at 116 Garden State Parkway in Holmdel, New Jersey, or at 2936 Marti Lane in Montgomery, Alabama, to name but a few of the thousand centers that were supposed to suffice for testing three hundred and thirty million Americans.

Congress had required the President to assemble a National Testing Strategy by mid-May. His first move was to gather a group of expert advisors. The crack team consisted of political hacks who were not by any stretch of the imagination experts in public health policy. Our Treasury Secretary Steve Mnuchin for example had been a Hollywood executive producer with a track record of tremendous box office flops like "Black Mass," "In the Heart of the Sea," and ironically, "Rules Don't Apply." President Trump's "experts" adopted a "Don't call us and we won't call you" plan, which was a solution akin to IDPH's response to COVID-19 calls of inquiry.

By the end of May, our "national testing strategy," by which I mean the federal plan to tell state governors that they are on their own, had in three months accomplished the testing of sixteen million, seven hundred and ninety-four thousand, one hundred and eighty-two of us[1], roughly five percent of our population

At that rate, in five short years, state health officials will have tested our entire population, or rather, the percent of our people who had not died because they were never tested for COVID-19. Of those tests, twelve percent were confirmed as positive cases. If we extrapolate from that small sample, we can assume that when all is said and done, if all Americans were tested for COVID-19, there would be nearly forty million positive cases, with elderly, infirmed, and diverse ethnic populations bearing the brunt of more than a million Coronavirus fatalities.

No unified testing strategy evolved because President Trump did not believe the Coronavirus would affect the red states which voted for him in 2016. He came to that conclusion when the pandemic spiked in New York and New Jersey. His people were not dying, and by that unholy pragmatism, it did not matter how many people who were not his supporters perished. If the pandemic had first spiked in Texas or Florida, then perhaps Jared Kushner and President Trump might have decided to approach the pandemic as a political problem which could only be resolved by instituting a national testing strategy. By the time those red states became hotspots, the pandemic was uncontrollable.

When my phone rang at 10 a.m. on April 9, I reached for my notebook and leaflet and answered my call from "Test Results." I spoke the first words that came to my mind, which were, "Wow, I'm glad you called." Expecting a more traditional "hello," the woman asked who I was. I said, "that's what I was going to ask you." I gave her my name, my date of birth, and my phone number which she had just called, but she did not identify herself. Instead she inquired if I still had the "Test Results" handout I was given at the Community Based Testing Site. When I responded that I was looking at it, she said, "Let's read through it together." I asked which part should we read—the part that says "**If you test *positive*"** at the top, or the part that says "**If you test *negative*"** at the bottom of the page. My heart throbbed at the bottom of my feet when she replied, "The top."

Not wanting to draw a hasty conclusion, and sounding much like the dullard she expected to encounter on most of her calls, I asked, "Are you telling me I tested positive?" I was prepared for her answer, and when she told me "'Yes" in a matter-of-fact tone, I had a number of questions at the ready. I asked "What is the reliability and validity of the test? What is the standard deviation?" I thought those were reasonable questions that any poor soul would have in mind when, like the condemned convict on death row awaiting a call from the governor's office to halt an imminent execution, we tried in vain to wiggle our way out of the handcuffs and chest bands which bound us to our seat in the gas chamber.

I was disappointed but not surprised to hear her say, "It's reliable." She may not have understood the meaning of the term "validity," because she ignored that part of my question. When I asked her for the data supporting her offhand conclusion that "it's reliable," she told me with fine-tuned impatience "You can get tested again."

She then directed me to look at the "keep your entire household home" line. The following bullet points were listed under that general topic:

- Most cases can be cared for at home.

- Do not go to the hospital to seek care unless you have a medical emergency.

- Do not go to work. Notify your employer of your positive test result.

- **Continue to monitor your symptoms at home as described on the opposite side.**

- Seek medical attention if you develop ANY of the following:

The symptoms listed under that subcategory were identical to the ones previously stated twice on the other pages of the leaflets. As she read through those symptoms I contemplated telling her that the IDPH needed to add more symptoms to the list, because many people who read their leaflet would fly off the handle when they saw that the symptoms they manifested weren't common or possible symptoms. I would have liked to hear her confirm that weird dreams such as mine and my absentmindedness had often been reported. Since she was in the middle of a process that she probably completed a hundred times a day, I did not interrupt her again. I saved my questions until her rote recital ended.

She next came to the blue boxes in the middle of the page. The question posed in the light-blue box on the left asked me, "**What should you expect?**" Technically, the first item listed,

- Most people experience minor symptoms such as fever and cough

was the only expectation defined by the Department of Public Health. The two bullet points which followed consisted of a suggestion and a sobering disclosure:

- Over-the-counter medications that lesson symptoms of fever and cough may help. It is important to get rest and drink plenty of fluids.

- There is currently no vaccine or medication to treat or prevent COVID-19.

She did not wait for me to respond when she read the navy-blue box on the right, which asked me "**When does home isolation end?**" I thought hers was a rhetorical question; its obvious answer was "the minute an ambulance arrives to take me to the hospital." But the U.S. Public Health Service, which I believe was "a wholly-owned subsidiary of Hadden Industries,"[2] provided the following guidelines:

- If you test positive for COVID-19, stay home and limit contact with others until:

    — You have been fever-free for at least 3 days without using medicine that reduces fever

  AND

    — Your symptoms have improved

  AND

    — At least 7 days have passed since your symptoms first appeared

- You need to consult your employer prior to returning to work.

There should have been a penalty imposed for anyone who ended self-quarantine without meeting these basic guidelines, but I realized such a practice would never happen in our country. Since states were free to enter

Phase, One, Two, or Three whenever they saw fit and without having penalties imposed for violating the CDC's "suggestions," then anyone lacking scruples could exhibit a similar "law of the land" disregard for the health of everyone with whom they came into contact.

For reasons I could not fathom, my IDPH representative felt compelled to read to me the final section of the page. Located above the final banner telling everyone to visit the Coronavirus government website was the section addressing people who had tested negatively. That section of the leaflet included these pieces of advice for those lucky contestants:

- You are probably not infected at this time. However, you could have been exposed and test positive later. You must continue to practice all protective measures to keep yourself and others negative.

- As long as the virus that causes COVID-19 is spreading in your community, continue to follow recommendations to protect yourself, including:

  — practice social distancing, wash your hands often, avid touching your face, and avoid social gatherings according to local guidance.

- Follow guidance from your healthcare provider and your state and local health departments.

I could have sat there all morning with my phone to my ear and read along with her, like bored eighth-graders listening to a classmate, the one with a with a third-grade reading ability, struggle to recite the textbook passage that they had finished reading to themselves five minutes earlier. I decided that a more fruitful course of action would be to put my phone on speaker and to prepare my Ninja Nuke while she plowed her way through the predetermined course of the call.

I had developed what I believed was a quick and efficient process for making my Ninja Nuke. First, forty-two almonds became my substrate. Then came the carrot, followed by the tablespoons of flaxseed meal, topped with a delicate flavoring of turmeric and finely-ground black pepper. The romaine was included after I chopped and added the celery. I crammed the ingredients into the container as far down as humanly possible, and I covered the mix with a smashed banana, as though I were putting frosting on a cake. I left a small gap on one side of the container, which would serve as a tunnel to deliver the apple juice quickly into depths of the vessel. If I did not provide that marginal opening, it would take forever for the apple juice to trickle its way down to the bottom of the receptacle, and there was always hell to pay if I was too impatient to wait for a sufficient amount of juice to filter its way through the ingredients to allow for a proper fill. A Ninja Nuke that was not correctly diluted would provide me with a durable substance I could use to spackle any imperfections in my living room wall. I had also learned the hard way that I should open the half-gallon of apple juice *before* refrigerating it. When I forgot to do that, some immutable law of quantum physics dictated that an adjustable wrench would be needed to apply enough torque to unscrew the plastic top of the jug. I felt proud that I had successfully parlayed the sum of the knowledge that I had accumulated in my life to allow me to discern the most efficacious way to master these morning elixir nuances.

After the blade assembly was tightly attached to the container and with the machine on ready mode, five applications of the pulse button and seven seconds each in the low, medium, and high speeds would result in emulsification at a desirable level of consistency. The mixture would be a little gritty because of the fine particles of almond nut residue that could not be eliminated by my machine, but there were no chunks of any food product that might cause me to choke. The degree of tightness of the blade assembly seal was critical; any laziness on that front caused a seeping or spraying of the mixture on the body of the machine and often on my kitchen countertop, window, and ceiling.

People often question why it will take so long to find a vaccine for the Coronavirus. I could easily understand why creating a vaccine would take more than a year. It had taken me over a week to discover how best to facilitate a simple kinetic process like making a Ninja Nuke. Assembling the raw materials that scientists needed to research a vaccine was probably more difficult than buying the Kirkland brand of almonds at Costco and counting out forty-two of them. The gadgets that they used to accomplish their goal were probably more sophisticated than my Nutri Ninja, which likely would extend their learning curve. Calibrating an ocular micrometer required more expertise than hand-tightening the blade assembly of the Nutri Ninja, and they most likely had to push more than four buttons. Their end goal was bound to be more elusive than it was for me trying to find a happy medium of consistency, somewhere between thin as a rail and thick as a brick. Give scientists all the time they need, I say; theirs is not a task to be taken lightly.

I was anxious for her to finish her narration because then it would be my turn, my one and only shot at receiving from the Illinois Department of Public Health the expert guidance that was not included on the three sides of my leaflets. I wanted the upper number of a COVID-19 induced temperature to be specified. I needed a further explication of the meaning of "difficult to wake up." I wondered what constituted a minor-league cough versus a Chicago Cubs Wrigley Field quality cough. I did not expect her to be Sigmund Freud, but I wanted to know if other patients had experienced strange dreams or nightmares. Should I waterboard Gatorade to make sure that I was drinking "plenty of fluids?" What should I do when considerably more than seven days have passed since my symptoms first appeared and they have not improved? What if I got a fever seventy-one hours after my last fever? Would that be close enough for me to consider myself fever-free? When would the contact tracing start? Is President Trump ever going to get off his fat ass and do something for us? How do I get out of this chickenshit outfit?

I could tell she wanted me to answer "no" when she finished her litany. With a sigh she added her obligatory epitaph, "Do you have any questions?" I asked her each of the above questions except for the last two, which a sense of decorum prohibited me from voicing. I did not receive a single scoff or rueful groan or an exasperated "Are you crazy?" in reply, but I was sure eyerolling was involved each time she told me "You need to consult with your medical professional." When I calmly inquired, "Can I speak to your supervisor?" she informed me that if I had any further questions, I should go online to the DPH website. Having traveled down that path before, I thanked her for her time and told her the only thing that came to mind, which was my equivalent of "so long honey babe, where I'm bound I can't tell." Before she disconnected the line, I heard her talking to a colleague about dining options for lunch that afternoon. To my knowledge, that was the beginning and end of contact tracing.

I followed her advice and called my doctor. He told me that I was his twenty-fourth patient who had reported a positive test. He was concerned about my symptoms but did not suggest hospitalization. A better course of treatment, he said, would consist of monitoring symptoms and to let him know each day how I was progressing. He knew my medical history and was aware of my proclivity to treat illnesses holistically. He said that black tea would be more effective than green tea for breaking up lung mucus and he suggested that natural licorice might also help achieve that same effect. He admitted this was a horrible disease and encouraged me to stay true to my routine. Most importantly, he said I should not be dismayed by the duration of the symptoms or by the overall length of time it may take to recover. I felt invigorated after our discussion. It gave me the emotional boost I needed after learning that my test was positive.

I had waited so long to get a test, and now that I had the result I had expected to receive, it was time to take stock of my situation. I recognized that this was now officially a matter of life or death, and a concise inventory of what I had experienced so far was required if I were to map a successful strategy for beating COVID-19.

I had slowly climbed my way up to one hundred and forty-five sit ups a day before breakfast, and I could tolerate the caffeine in three cups of tea after my Ninja Nuke. I noticed that I experienced a more frequent and violent dry cough at two times of the day—after eating, and halfway between breakfast and dinner. I came to realize that eating produced saliva that tickled my throat and esophagus, which would seem to account for the coughing after meals. The only explanation I had for the midday bout was that my body was short of the energy it needed to allow my immune system to function optimally. I concluded that besides providing enough energy to exercise, a sufficient intake of food was necessary to fight the deleterious effect that the cytokine storm had on my lungs.

I had not yet determined why my cough had remained dry for so long and why more coughing resulted when standing or sitting than when reclining. I was glad that was the pattern, though, because it would be horrible to lay in bed and cough all night. Headaches and chills were enough of a challenge to sleeping soundly, and I would invariably twist and turn before I passed out from exhaustion.

Sonia had a major complaint in that department. She was used to me reclining on my left side, with my left arm outstretched under a blanket, and remaining there for the night. This position allowed her to rest her body against my upper arm and to place her head on the inside of my elbow, with her front feet outstretched so she could claw affectionately into the top of my hand for an hour before she fell asleep. She could not understand why I could not stay put and let her sleep peacefully. She resigned herself to a spot at the foot of my bed where she could remain undisturbed by my fidgeting.

I found that standing upright while coughing was a dangerous posture. Coughing caused my lungs to hurt but coughing while standing caused my whole body to jerk. Adapting to sneezing fits was also challenging. One day I twisted my right knee when I sneezed unexpectedly while standing, and I was not sure when the soreness would disappear. After that injury I learned to seek an appropriate position when I sensed that I was about to sneeze or cough. I would lean against my refrigerator if it were nearby, or I would sit on the floor. I was becoming more limber from doing my sit ups, but all my muscles ached when I tried to stand after coughing while seated. It was a lamentable state of being. I had descended several rungs down the ladder from the height of yoga flexibility I had attained six weeks ago. I hoped to regain that proficiency after I had circumvented the rigamarole of this disease.

Chills came in waves, and I found it helpful to add a sweater, a vest, and sometimes a scarf and ski cap to my daily wardrobe. Although the room temperature was set at eighty degrees, I never felt warm enough, except when I stood in a steam-filled bathroom after a hot shower. I did four minutes of breathing exercises while showering, and the combination of those exercises and the steam made my lungs felt less stressed. Those were the moments of release that bolstered my resolve to do all I could to feel better.

I would cough to the point of gagging after inhaling five breaths of steam rising from my uncovered pot of green tea, but once that had occurred a few times, I noticed that the wheezing sound when I exhaled with force had diminished. I never deviated from my breathing exercise routine; I feared that I would develop lung fibrosis if I were not vigilant, and I knew that fibrosis could not be reversed.

I encountered one more episode of middle of the night breathing impairment. I followed the only course of treatment I knew, which was to try to relax, and watch television while sitting. I stayed in that position until I felt more certain that autonomous breathing would return if I laid down.

I was in a quandary over how long to sit up before I could safely attempt to sleep. I noticed a phenomenon that I should have recognized the previous time I was unable to breathe. After an hour of sitting while watching two <u>Green Acres</u> reruns, I attempted to yawn but could not. After another hour, my eyes grew heavy during an infomercial for Nugenix and I yawned. I was pleased to discover I was able to yawn fully. I felt I then had found a reliable standard to employ to tell me when it was safe for me to attempt sleep; when I found I could yawn normally, I knew I would breathe normally if I slept. Someone else might have figured out the correlation sooner than I did, but since I am not a stupid person, I could only conclude that my ability to recognize a solution had been waylaid by my fear of not being able to breathe.

I wondered if President Trump struggled with a similar psychology. Did his fear of not being re-elected preclude him from noticing that over a hundred thousand Americans had died needlessly on his watch? I had no one to ask "When is it safe to go back to sleep?" at four o'clock in the morning, but the President had cadres of inept consultants and spineless advisors whose job it was to tell him to open his eyes. They were too afraid to alert him to the specifics of what he failed to grasp because our President does not countenance criticism or bad news. No one in his circle dared to incur his wrath and risk their chance of returning to office after the November election. His Cabinet wanted another four years on the job, and his Congressional following wanted to ride into office on his coattails.

My temperature, which I tracked four times a day, was stable at one hundred and one degrees. I had been taking a low dose aspirin four times a day. Now that I had a test positive to add to my resume' I decided that in a day or two I would perform my experiment to document what happened to my temperature without aspirin intake. Procrastination gave me time to consider all variables. I would need to limit my fluid intake when I went cold turkey. I would do some research to determine what was a risky but marginally safe maximum temperature to attain and how long should it be prolonged.

171

If I was going to avoid aspirin and liquids and allow my fever do whatever it wanted to do, I needed first to attain some level of confidence that the process would not backfire on me, that I would not suffer additional injuries from having sustained too high a temperature for too long of a timeframe. Before undertaking this endeavor, I also needed to determine the quickest, safe way to reduce body temperature if my fever did not break of its own accord.

I would not have considered the process I was now contemplating to be a prudent course of action if I had not been in the high-risk category of COVID-19 patients and if the symptoms I had been experienced had not been prolonged. I was certain that most people taking note of this behavior would judge this radical action to be a dangerous folly, but I guessed that those people holding that contrary opinion were not COVID-19 victims and were not in immediate danger of dying. I would make a final determination after weighing all the pros and cons, but my instinct was to perform this therapy sooner rather than later.

My emotional support system had been limited to the companionship Sonia provided, which I felt might not be sufficient to see me through to the finish. I texted my Countryside friends, and they were sympathetic to my plight. After I informed them of this news, not a day would pass without one of them texting me, wondering how I was doing. One of them described how he would say a Hail Mary and would tell ten people to do the same, and those persons would tell ten more people, and so on. They offered to purchase and to bring me any supplies I needed; they would leave what they bought at my doorstep. I thanked them in a text and told them I was okay for now, but if any needs arose, I would contact them. I told two of my cousins about my positive test. They both offered prayers and good wishes. One of them sent me a box of thyme tea, and I included a thyme teabag with my black tea each time I made a pot. Although thyme tea was not an antiviral agent, it possessed antibacterial properties which would help keep my weakened lungs from contracting bacterial pneumonia.

I decided to be more aggressive with my Ninja Nuke and increase my dose of turmeric to one teaspoon. I discovered that such a large quantity could be tolerated only if the amount was incrementally increased. If done too quickly, gastrointestinal distress and nausea were the sure results. The half-teaspoon of pepper did not need to be increased; turmeric absorption was guaranteed with that minimum amount of pepper. To keep the turmeric from staining the heavy, clear-plastic Nutri Ninja container, it was necessary to rinse it thoroughly after each use. Emulsified liquid tended to stick to the container's sides, and to eliminate bacteria from forming in a nutrient-rich environment, a thorough rinsing with hot water and scrubbing were required after each use. The blades were quite sharp, and care had to be taken when that assembly was washed each day. I did not use soap on either item because I did not want to drink leftover dish detergent as part of each morning's marginally palatable Ninja Nuke. I was grateful that my COVID-19 symptoms did not include nausea. I attributed my lack of nausea to adequate hydration.

I gradually increased fluid intake until I drank a gallon of liquid a day. The total would consist of apple juice, tea, diet cherry soda, Gatorade, and water that I would flavor with powered lemonade or Tang. The one liquid I no longer drank was alcohol. The ounce of Crown Royal I had consumed at Countryside on March 10 was the last spirit I had imbibed. Sure, I would have liked to have a beer or a Canadian Club with ginger ale every now and then, but I felt it was a luxury that I could not afford to embrace. I did not want to divert my weakened immune system from its goal of rebuilding itself by asking it to please spend a few minutes to take care of these alcohol molecules that I am recklessly and unnecessarily sending your way. The Coronavirus had a demonstrated negative effect on heart and liver functions. I thought it wise to refrain from having a Blue Moon with an orange slice in case my liver or heart was fighting a higher-ground battle. My intake of vitamin C pills and grapefruit juice did not need the marginal, additional assistance that an orange slice would provide.

I remained unconvinced about a possible beneficial interaction between medical cannabis and COVID-19, so I continued to avoid its use. The consultants at the dispensary could not substantiate industry claims that CBD had medicinal properties to help me fight the Coronavirus.

I stopped drinking most liquids by 7 p.m. I had found that it was extremely frustrating once I had fallen into sleep to force myself to get up to visit the bathroom. My goal each night was to sleep as soundly as possible and to stay in bed as late as possible each morning. My symptoms worsened when I varied from that routine.

Because I felt I was meeting the IDPH guideline of drinking plenty of fluid each day, I could not understand why on some nights I would find myself suddenly encountering severe leg and foot cramps. I did not know if cramps were resulting from as simple a cause as an unfortunate choice of sleeping posture or if they signaled CIDP rolling up its formidable sleeves and going to work, as had happened in the past. I decided to regard the syndrome as "Covid Cramps," with an amorphous cause of unpredictable severity. My therapy for cramps was to lean into the cramp, to stretch the front of my foot upward if my arch was cramping or to stand and lean into a calf cramp with my leg bent, to stretch the affected tendon. I had learned not to worry about symptoms that I did not consider to be life threatening because at some point they would disappear and would cause no permanent damage.

Objectively, I found it startling that I would regard so many issues that might have previously sent me to a doctor's office for a consult as no more than minor inconveniences. Whenever I suffered from sciatica pain, I would call my doctor, describe the symptom to him, and rate the level of pain. I currently had been faithful to my commitment to perform an increasing number of sit ups each day, but still, my spending so much time in bed exacted its inevitable price, which was experiencing an ongoing series of twisted side and back muscles. I could not sleep very well on my back, and stress would occur if I moved my legs too quickly when sleeping in a fetal position.

To alleviate the pain, I applied generous amounts of Biofreeze to the affected areas, which seemed to be the most effective over-the-counter topical anesthetic. I found that the roll-on variety was easier to apply, and it would permit application to places like my upper back that I could not otherwise reach. I kept a tube of it at bedside, but I no longer used the gel variety. I had learned that using my fingertips to apply the gel, which deadened nerves perhaps more effectively than did the roll-on type, was not a good idea if I planned to play guitar. Practicing for the ten minutes while trying not to cough was a big enough challenge; not being able to feel the strings at the fourteenth fret with my fingertips, for example, would have made the exercise pointless.

Because my cough had remained dry for so long, I toyed with the concept of using an expectorant. I did not want to inculcate too dry of a lung environment and decided to stick with the breathing exercises I was doing with a damp washcloth and hope for the best.

I would have liked to have been able to hike a mile in each direction to the nearest grocery store, a Shop and Save on Nagle Avenue, to purchase more romaine, celery, carrots, bananas, a pound of thinly sliced prosciutto, and vegetables for dinner. I also needed more soda, juice, and Gatorade. I was confident I had enough stamina to enable a walk of that distance, and I could stop along the way in the park to marvel at squirrels searching for nuts, to observe robins hunting for worms, and frankly to see other humans interact. None of that was possible because I was self-quarantined. I called a friend and asked him to please pick up those items for me next time he was shopping. He was glad to help and delivered the items two hours later. He buzzed me on the intercom and said he would make the same delivery a week later.

I thanked him and relaxed a bit. I was glad he anticipated my future need because I was not sure I would be fit as a fiddle in a week's time. When he asked how it felt to sleep so long each day, I described for him the different type of sleep cycle that I was experiencing. Sleeping had become a mechanical exercise, not a restful activity. Each morning I would awake wondering if my health had improved or declined overnight. I told him that sleeping so long led to a desire to sleep longer, that each morning it took an hour to regain a sense of confidence that today would be better than the previous day, that today would be the last day I would feel so bad. It was a longer and more complex answer than he most likely was expecting to hear, but he told me to hang in there and he would stop by again next week.

I had started eating protein for lunch, which consisted of an ounce of prosciutto and cheese. The meat portion of that respite came to an end one day when I noticed Sonia avoiding the cheese but sniffing the prosciutto on my plate. She did not try to eat it, because it was too large of a lump, and her congested condition prohibited her from remaining too long in a head-down position. I had elevated her dry and wet food bowls on three books to raise them closer to her body level. I tried the same with the prosciutto, but it was too new a set of circumstances to succeed. She sniffed at the prosciutto and walked away.

Whenever she was reluctant to eat wet food, I stood her in my lap. When she placed her front paws on my shoulder, I held a pinch of the food in front of her face so that she could smell what was coming her way. Enticed by the scent, when she opened her mouth, I placed the morsel of food at the back of her tongue, and she swallowed it readily.

I tore the prosciutto into small pieces. When Sonia assumed her eating position on my chest, I shoved tender bits of that twelve dollar a pound deli meat into her mouth. She ate a tablespoon of prosciutto, and when it was gone, she hopped down, drank some water, and looked at me quizzically, as if to say, "Why didn't you think of that sooner, you dummy?" For as long as it lasted, prosciutto replaced all varieties of Fancy Feast as her favorite meal.

I was happy with my own dinner menu, which consisted of a pasta and vegetable variation each night. I never grew tired of it and I figured that by utilizing a consistent diet I could control caloric intake. I was forced to rethink this policy a few weeks later when I found out that COVID-19 patients who were obese or who had Type One or Two diabetes had an extraordinarily high mortality rate. I was not obese or diabetic, but I did not want to develop either conditions due to an uncontrolled intake of carbs from lasagna, carbonara, and tagliatelle. I decided to limit each portion to four ounces of uncooked pasta. I found that when warming leftover pasta in my microwave, it was helpful to add olive oil before reheating. This way, I avoided turning the entrée into a sticky pile of congealed goo after three minutes at a high setting.

The results of the diabetes study also led me to reexamine my practice of enjoying the dessert buffet of cookies and sweets to which I looked forward every night. Even if I could not taste the sweetness, I remembered that everything I was eating was quite yummy. Once more, a memory of a sensation replaced the real thing. Since my taste buds had fallen asleep, limiting my intake of sweets was not difficult.

With my updated inventory of aches and pains, chills and ills, hopeful theories, adequate and inadequate supplies, and proposed remedies in hand, I felt prepared to battle the Coronavirus. I would remain open to any new strategies that a stray thought or an errant, middle of the night awareness might engender.

One such thought occurred to me a few nights later. I knew I had to conserve energy. I also knew I had to find an indoor activity that would be energizing. Beginning a home improvement project like re-tiling my kitchen floor was too exhausting a prospect to contemplate. I need an exercise that would improve my balance, one that I could sustain for a half-hour a day without a deleterious side effect.

I looked through my stack of exercise dvd's and I found one entitled <u>Introductory Yoga</u> which would fit the bill. If I proceeded slowly, I should be able to manage Warrior One and Warrior Two in short order. I would not push too hard and I would not compare my current lack of skills to any prior efficiency I had attained. I would be happy if I had a better sense of balance in a week. Yoga practice might also reduce cramping, which would be a delightful byproduct.

I dusted off my copy of <u>Getting Well Again</u> by Dr. O. Carl Simonton. His book emphasized the importance of creating strong mental and physical imagery when fighting cancer. His instructions which were geared for creating tumor-fighting imagery could be easily retooled for fighting COVID-19. Simonton encouraged his patients to draw pictures of how they saw their fight unfolding. He also stressed the importance of mediation, which I equated with prayer. His book indicated one more line of attack in a multi-faceted approach to fighting COVID-19. It offered a psychological approach that would become an essential part of my daily playbook.

I followed the IDPH guideline and informed my employers that I had tested positively. It was not necessary for me to do so because I had typically worked from my home office and my employers had already been closed their offices in compliance with social distancing orders.

The term "social distancing" was not a term created during the Coronavirus pandemic. Its use grew out of the study of Proxemics, which was a traditional form of analyzing human comfort zones when engaging others in discussions, when standing in line at the Department of Motor Vehicles, or when chatting up an attractive woman at the Morrison Roadhouse. Its first pandemic application occurred in 2003 during the Severe Acute Respiratory Syndrome outbreak. Its use resurfaced during the 2006 Avian Flu epidemic, but it did not become "a buzzword of these strange times"[3] until the National Institute of Health and the Center for Disease Control used the term to describe a Novel Coronavirus mitigation strategy.

With tragically little understanding of its meaning, President Trump used the "social distancing" term as a sound bite, capitalizing on it shock appeal. He then ignored the term and its applications, with one important exception. He made damned sure that each press corps member that gathered in the Romper Room or the Gypsy Rose Lee Garden for one of his ill-fated Task Force Briefings or ludicrous press conferences was separated from one another by at least six feet, because this spacing would limit the number of reporters that could cause him problems, asking pesky questions such as, "Mr. President, what data do you have to support that statement?" or "What were you thinking, Sir, when you told Michael Atkinson to go fuck himself?" Social distancing was fine for reporters; meanwhile, our President stood elbow to coughing elbow with whomever he commanded to take center stage with him. I promised myself that when the Admiral Theater on Lawrence Avenue re-opened, for example, I would abide by its social distancing suggestions if I chose to visit the establishment, and I would not accept any twenty-five dollar lap dances offered by any of the Admiral's nude dancers who did not wear face coverings.

My daily routine helped me to not lose track of the hours passing in a day, but I no longer had a clear sense of days passing. No differentiation between a work week and weekend existed. Sundays and holidays distinguished themselves solely by a lack of mail delivery, but because on most days I did not get any mail, that frail distinction disappeared. Because it no longer mattered to me if it was Monday or Friday by the calendar, weeks began to blend seamlessly.

I watched at least two hours of news each evening, and I continued to take note of the various Presidential gaffs and ignominies with which we were blighted each day. If I were invited to the White House and could perform one song for the President, it would be "Dirty Boulevard" from Lou Reed's New York album. The lines "Your poor huddled masses, let's club 'em to death/And get it over with" would not resonate well with him, but they summed up his attitude toward Coronavirus victims.

The lyric also characterized his actions toward individuals brazen enough to protest peacefully near Pennsylvania Avenue when he wanted to visit St.

John's Episcopal Church, not for prayer or to profess a belief system of any sort, but for a photo opportunity. He held a Bible in his hand with his arm outstretched, as though the Good Book was a flag to be waved, a talisman signifying a pledge of Higher allegiance, one which he has never fulfilled. His reckless choices, like the one to militarize Washington, DC, and previous comments of his, such as "Why are we having all these people from shithole countries come here?"[4] illustrate his lack of love of his neighbor and his larger, blatant contempt for any Old or New Testament teaching.

It is too bad that in less than one short term in office President Trump has simultaneously failed to demonstrate a love of God and to desecrate the symbology of our flag. If he had acknowledged either concept as sacrosanct, if he had been motivated by a sense of moral obligation to fight the pandemic, hundreds of thousands of us might still be alive. It is tragically coincidental that the pandemic occurred while Mr. Trump was President. No other administration could have handled the Coronavirus pandemic more poorly, and we would not have borne so heavy a burden of losses of life if we had been blessed with a different gatekeeper. Unfortunately, with each passing day, I watched the Coronavirus become more mature and lethal, while each of President Trump's decisions demonstrated less maturity and equal virulence.

For no apparent reason, on the nights of April 12 and April 13, I experienced a nasty set of chills. My temperature with aspirin intake rose to one hundred and two. My teeth chattered for ten minutes at a time. An hour later, after I had completely covered myself with two blankets, I felt extremely overheated. My heart rate was elevated by fifty percent. I ditched the blankets, in a cycle that continued throughout the two nights. Because I was not coughing and my breathing was regular, I waited it out each night by praying.

When I felt overheated I envisioning peaceful scenes, recalling the tranquil solitude I felt when I skied Via Lattea's slopes in the Piedmont region of Northern Italy; when I hiked in Yellowstone on a late-autumn afternoon; when I watched the snow-covered mountaintops pass by my window as I rode a train through the east end of the Golden Pass between Luzern and Interlaken; and when I marveled at a marmot's funny gait as he scampered across my cool, mossy trail in Olympic National Park in early spring. I do not know if these thoughts reduced my temperature, but they did lead me to the edge of sleep.

My dreams were not always disjointed, but I remember that for those two nights, they were scattered and deranged. In one doolally of a rapid eye movement session I was concomitantly on the cusp of making an earth-shaking scientific discovery; finding a winning scratch-off ticket in the parking lot of a retail store like Wieboldt's that has been closed for the past forty-five years; and worrying that I would not defuse an atomic devise in time to save the world from doom.

After the second night I decided it was time to go World War Z on my fever. If I took no action, I believed that in time my waking, cognitive abilities would resemble my dream-state and I would become as nutty as a fruitcake. I could continue to abate my temperature with aspirin, but that action would not kill the Coronavirus. I had done due diligence and found that tolerating a temperature of one hundred and four for an hour would not result in brain damage, and a cold shower was the best way to reduce my body temperature quickly.

At 9 p.m. on April 14 my temperature was one hundred and two, and I did not take any aspirins. By midnight it had risen two degrees, and perspiration beaded my forehead. Between 2 a.m. and 3 a.m. I remained at a steady one hundred and five. Had it increased, I would have swallowed aspirins and taken that shower, but the thermometer's digital display did not flicker beyond that number. By 4 a.m. my pajamas, sheets, and pillowcase were soaked in sweat. I resisted the urge to throw off the blankets, stand on my balcony, and stay there until the sweat on my forehead froze. I was ready to cheer and uncork a bottle of Dom Perignon when at 5 a.m. I took my temperature and saw that it had settled on the century mark. I took a warm shower, put on a clean pair of pajamas, and apologized to Sonia for all the ruckus, explaining that what had happened was perfectly natural, no need for her to look askance at me.

I believe she understood on a basic level that what she had witnessed with her night vision over the past few hours resembled the existential threats she faced which had cause her to spend three of her nine lives. Her first brush with death had come when she had been abandoned beneath her previous home. Her second close encounter had occurred when she nearly died of respiratory failure before I realized I could treat her with the decongestant. Her third life was spent a week before The Sneeze. She was breathing normally when I went to sleep, but at 130 a.m. I awoke and recognized that I could not hear her gentle snoring. She was laying on her side at the foot of my bed, and her tail did not move when I touched it. Her legs did not change position when I petted her stomach, and she moved her head away from me when I petted her there. Her breathing was raspy and weak, and she made no throat clearing noises when I rubbed the side of her head. I panicked and cried. I was afraid her little motor would stop running and I would lose her. I put my head next to hers and listened. After a while I thought her breathing sounded more regular. I stayed awake in that position for hours and fell asleep when I heard her beginning to snore.

I wondered what she was dreaming during that episode. I know that she experiences REMs and that the electrical activity occurring in her brain while sleeping closely resembles the sleeping activity in the brains of other mammals like humans. My guess is that she was reliving her favorite activity of that day, which was playing with the end of my phone's recharging cord as I dangled it toward and away from her, letting her capture and chew it for as long as she found it interesting. Perhaps she was having fun chasing the moth that had invaded her space by entering through my patio door. If that was the case, I envied her ability to block out any unpleasant memory, such as the daily decongestant dose, and recall only the fun moments in her life. I wished that I would not have to wait until November elections to remove bad memories from my dreaming and waking states.

For whatever reason, my fever never returned, but I still had difficulty breathing, and I wondered for the hundredth time if coughing was exacerbating breathing difficulties by hurting my lungs, or if coughing was a sign that I was on the mend. I looked forward to the soothing menthol contained in each of my oral anesthetics. I realized I could not go through the rest of my life as a Halls' Honey Lemon Cough Drop addict, but I did not know how to prevent that outcome.

I revisited the topic of lung functions a week later, when an Opinion piece in the Sunday, April 20 New York Times caught my eye. It was written by Dr. Richard Levitan, who was an emergency department physician. He described what he had witnessed when attending to patients for a ten-day period at Bellevue Hospital in New York City. He noticed that "almost all the E.R. patients had Covid pneumonia."[5] He stated that with "patients on whom we did CT scans because they were injured in falls, we coincidentally found Covid pneumonia. Elderly patients who had passed out for unknown reasons and a number of diabetic patients were found to have it."

Those patients "did not report any sensation of breathing problems, even though their chest X-rays showed diffuse pneumonia and their oxygen was below normal." He developed a theory "that Covid pneumonia initially causes a form of oxygen deprivation we call "silent hypoxia"—'silent' because of its insidious, hard-to-detect nature." He noticed that "when Covid pneumonia first strikes, patients don't feel short of breath, even as their oxygen levels fall. And by the time they do, they have alarmingly low oxygen levels and moderate-to-severe pneumonia...Normal oxygen saturation for most persons at sea level is 94 to 100 percent; Covid pneumonia patients I saw had oxygen saturations as low as 50 percent."

Those same individuals "had been sick for a week or so with fever, cough, upset stomach and fatigue, but they only became short of breath the day they came to the hospital. Their pneumonia had clearly been going on for days, but by the time they felt they had to go to the hospital, they were often already in critical condition." Dr. Levitan wrote that "a vast majority of Covid pneumonia patients I met had remarkably low oxygen saturations at triage—seemingly incompatible with life—but they were using their cellphones as we put them on monitors. Although breathing fast, they had relatively minimal apparent distress, despite dangerously low oxygen levels and terrible pneumonia on chest X-rays."

He explained the incongruity of low oxygen saturation not causing other symptoms in these terms: "The coronavirus attacks lung cells that make surfactant. This substance helps the air sacs in the lungs stay open between breaths and is critical to normal lung function. As the inflammation from Covid pneumonia starts, it causes the air sacs to collapse, and oxygen levels fall. Yet the lungs initially remain 'compliant,' not yet stiff or heavy with fluid. This means patients can still expel carbon dioxide—and without a buildup of carbon dioxide, patients do not feel short of breath." In this scenario, silent hypoxia causes "even more inflammation and more air sacs to collapse, and the pneumonia worsens until oxygen levels plummet. In effect, patients are injuring their own lungs by breathing harder and harder. Twenty percent of Covid pneumonia patients then go on to a second and deadlier phase of lung injury. Fluid builds up and the lungs become stiff, carbon dioxide rises, and patients develop acute respiratory failure." He believed that this syndrome "explains cases of Covid-19 patients dying suddenly after not feeling short of breath."

Dr. Levitan reported that "because Covid-19 overwhelmingly kills through the lungs" and "because so many patients are not going to the hospital until their pneumonia is already well advanced, many wind up on ventilators, causing shortages of the machines. And once on ventilators, many die." He did not mention that there was a final, more drastic method for extending life if venting failed produce a favorable response. As a last resort, an Extracorporeal Membrane Oxygenation device could be used, if one were available. The machine would pump blood through an artificial lung and back into the body, thereby skipping altogether the patient's ineffective lungs.

This ECMO process sounded extremely scary, and its existence and utilization heightened the plateau of fear I had reached by reading Dr. Levitan's description of venting. He explained that "Vented patients require multiple sedatives so that they don't buck the vent or accidentally remove their breathing tubes; they need intravenous and arterial lines, IV medicines and IV pumps. In addition to a tube in the trachea, they have tubes in their stomach and bladder. Teams of people are required to move each patient, turning them on their stomach and then their back, twice a day to improve lung function." The mechanics of venting led him to comment, "Avoiding the use of a ventilator is a huge win for both patient and the health care system." I assume he viewed ECMO as doubly problematic.

Dr. Levitan concluded that "detecting silent hypoxia early" would help avoid an expensive and complicated hospital stay, one which in many cases did not yield positive results. To achieve that early-detection goal, he offered this advice: "All patients who *have* tested positive for the coronavirus should have pulse oximetry monitoring for two weeks, the period during which Covid pneumonia typically develops."

Finally, after searching for more than a month, I had found an authoritative source which directly addressed the specific and predominant killing mechanism employed by the Coronavirus. I regretted that I had not purchased a pulse oximeter at CVS when I saw the rack of them on display, but I thought I could easily correct that mistake.

Once I got my finger into an oximeter, I would immediately check into the nearest ER if my level of oxygenation had edged toward fifty percent. Then I could take advantage of the earlier detection, non-ventilator forms of therapy Dr. Levitan had said would be in play. I met his criteria for early admission: I had been sick with fever, cough, and fatigue for more than a week; my lungs were compliant; I was injuring my lungs by breathing harder and harder; and I had tested positive.

His statement about damage caused by hard breathing hit home. I decided to continue with my breathing exercises but not to exhale as forcefully as I could, which had been my practice. Perhaps the wheezing sound I heard at the end of each exhalation resulted from putting too much pressure on my lungs. I wanted to exercise them and keep them as supple as I could, but I did not want to have an ischemic stroke by doing so. I would also proceed with caution when inhaling tea steam.

Drug stores had been deemed "essential services" and remained open during the part of social distancing called a "lockdown." The term "lockdown" bothered me. Its usage connoted scenes of prison cell doors slamming shut, of Spencer Tracey occupying his time turning big rocks into little ones in the 1932 Michael Curtiz film 20,000 Years in Sing Sing.

I had never been in a lockdown; it made the term "self-quarantine" sound easy-peasy. When it was over, if I escaped from a "lockdown," would the trauma of being locked down result in unwanted and detrimental emotional baggage? After all, things did not work out very well for Paul Muni at the end of Mervyn LeRoy's 1932 film I Am a Fugitive from a Chain Gang.

I wished that the term in vogue was economic "recess." A recess was a pleasant experience, describing the carefree time between penmanship and arithmetic classes when we frolicked on schoolyard baseball diamonds and dodged bullies trying to steal our lunch money. If Congress could take a time-out, certainly our economy was allowed a recess. All we had to do is avoid the use of that term's frightful kissing cousin, "recession," which, like "pandemic," was something "nobody bargained for, and only a lunatic wants."[6]

Drug stores had added delivery of goods to the line of services they could provide. I called CVS, then Walgreens, to purchase a reliable oximeter and to have the product delivered. Both stores were sold out of the item. Undaunted, I called the pharmacies of three close-by hospitals. None of them had the product in stock. I was told to try Walmart, which I did, with no better result forthcoming. I decided to wait until the next day to call every medical supply store in the Yellow Pages because, due to staff fur-loughing during the "lockdown," those businesses, like banks, were closed by 3 p.m. and re-opened at 9 a.m.

Working from a suspicion that I would strike out at Hook's Medical Supplies, Dr. Roberts' Med Shop, and Redman's Remedies, I looked online to see what the purchase of an oximeter from an unknown source would entail. Flagg's Farmacia promised to deliver an Andros Oximeter in four business days for thirty-nine dollars, plus tax. For Next-Day Air Service, I would need to add sixty dollars to the total. The surcharge was highway robbery. Since a packaged oximeter weighed less than a pound, R. Flagg was taking advantage of its desperate customers, attempting to capture a hefty revenue stream at our expense.

A better online option was O'Bannon's Balms, which guaranteed free ground delivery of a four-star Casper Oximeter in three days, for nineteen dollars and ninety-five cents. I ordered one as a Plan B, confident that I would get my hands on an honest-to-goodness, new, five-star oximeter by noon on Monday.

I admit I was frustrated by the complex task of obtaining a simple piece of medical equipment, an oximeter. It was difficult to gauge how desperate I would feel if I were a medical practitioner and I could not obtain the equipment I needed to protect myself when attempting to save the lives of COVID-19 patients. I wondered if I would I be brave enough to go to work knowing that by midday the limited supply of N-95 masks, face shields, and gowns would be exhausted. If I had that type of courage, would I continue to work a double shift when I understood the jeopardy into which I would be placed? My search for an oximeter brought those risks to light for me with striking clarity.

While I was in google mode, I thought it would be wise to do my research on how to operate an oximeter and how I should interpret the readings. I learned that the oximeter works best if it is attached to the middle finger of my dominant hand. But before I opened the non-hinged end and inserted my finger, I needed to clean its insides and my fingertip with a q-tip soaked in isopropyl. I was cautioned "**do not pour alcohol directly into the device,**" which made sense, because few electronic objects work well after being soaked in a liquid, a fact I discovered to be true a year ago when my phone inadvertently went through a cold water cycle in my washing machine.

Once the oximeter was cleaned, I should leave my finger inside it for a minute, because "readings will vary throughout the sixty seconds of the test." I should avoid movement and have my wrist "supported by a table or pillow." This was to avoid my "sustaining an injury due to the weight of the oximeter." Because my Seiko wristwatch weighed more than the oximeter, the likelihood of developing carpal tunnel syndrome caused by the six-ounce weight of the oximeter seemed to me to be minimal, but I would follow those directions because I was the amateur, and those instructions had been written and revised by professionals who made their livings by providing instructions to feeble-minded customers like myself.

To allow for variances within the gadget and within my metabolism, I should take multiple readings throughout the day. Fair enough, I thought, but I was worried that I had already introduced too many variables into what would otherwise appear to be a simple protocol. I should also keep a log of all findings for later analysis "by trained medical personnel." I admit that a doctor would be more knowledgeable about what oximeter results meant, but how hard could it be, I wondered, to interpret a numerical finding? A deep understanding of Newton's Second Law of Relativistic Dynamics and an awareness of the properties of dark matter were not required to determine if I was okay, borderline, or about to die based on oximeter readings.

I recognized the wisdom in the admonition, though, when I read that there was a further complication. The numbers which displayed both my pulse and my oxygenation level would be upside down. I was warned, "**do not confuse the two scores.**" While the chromo was reading the oxygen level of my finger, as an added value, it was also taking my pulse. I was informed that panic could be avoided if I did not confuse the two readings and assume, for example, that my oxygenation level was sixty-four, when that number was a reading of my pulse at rest.

Mindful of the various factors that would soon come into play, I developed a matrix to outline everything I should know when I tried to document my scores. At the offset I stupidly believed that this would be a simple process, but now I knew better. My matrix would remind me that I would have two scores, both of which would fluctuate throughout the sixty seconds of the test; that the scores should not be confused with one another; that all numbers would be upside-down; and that both scores would vary throughout the day. I understood that I would be devoting more time, energy, and concentration to a process I originally thought would be a slam-dunk, but nothing about COVID-19 was simple or easy to manage.

Now that I knew precisely how the oximeter apparatus would work, I realized it would be important to know exactly what the oxygenation number represented. After one quick google, I found the following table, which, rightly or wrongly, I assumed would answer my question of how I should interpret oximeter results:

Pulse Oximetry: What Do the Numbers Mean?

SpO2, %	PaO2, mm Hg	Oxygenation Status
95100	80100	Normal
9194	6080	Mild hypoxia
8690	5060	Moderate hypoxia
Less than 85	Less than 50	Severe hypoxia

I realized I would need professional help interpreting these types of results. Or conversely, I could stick with Dr. Levitan's easy-to-follow guideline. I was good if I was at ninety-four or above, and in trouble if it was lower than ninety-four.

It had taken a while for my knee to heal, but now that it was feeling better, I added gentle yoga to my daily regimen. I accomplished the two warrior poses, the chair, and a butterfly stretch without subsequent pain or injury. I needed to brace myself with my hands when I attempted a low lunge, and I could only manage a very shaky tree pose for a few seconds on either foot.

Patience equals success in yoga, and I would follow a program which would assuredly lead to improved balance.

By noon Monday I had concluded that medical supply stores carried all imaginable supplies except the one I needed. I called Meijers in Arlington Heights and a sympathetic pharmacist told me that he had heard that the Meijers at Stateline had their house brand of pulse oximeter in stock. I called that store and was told that they indeed had two on the shelf. I asked the person to please hold one for me, and he agreed.

My next problem was how to get to that Meijers store, which was in a suburb of Rockford called Love's Park. Normally this would be an easy two-hour jaunt by car, but since I was self-quarantined, I could not drive. I had never used Uber, but I found out I could use an Uber driver to drive to Love's Park, pick up my parcel, and bring it back to me. The service would cost about two hundred dollars.

I remembered that I had loaned a friend of mine a hundred dollars, and I called him and proposed that he could square his debt by running this errand. He lived in Elgin, which was about a third of the way to Love's Park, and he said he would do it if I added fifteen dollars for gas and tolls, plus the cost of the device. I agreed, and the problem was solved.

When he delivered the thingamajig he told me that instead of driving to the Wisconsin border, he had called the Meijers store in Plainfield, Illinois, where they had a surfeit of oximeters. He drove to the closer store and bought one off the shelf, on sale for twenty-nine dollars. He arrived an hour later. I buzzed him into the building, wrote him a check, and slid it under my door. He took the check and left the doohickey on the floor. I thanked him for his resourcefulness, because his not driving all the way to Love's Park resulted in me obtaining the prized oximeter more quickly.

I debated whether I should perform my first test before doing breathing exercises, when the results would not be artificially elevated by the exercises. The approach was appealing, because such a reading might be a truer index of my oxygenation level for most of the day. However, if I first exercised my lungs, I would obtain, in theory, the highest reading possible. I decided to cover both bases, and take the test before doing breathing exercises, and then repeat it a short time thereafter.

But I was getting ahead of myself. First, I had to remove the device from multiple layers of hard-shell plastic without damaging the contraption. Anyone who has ever attempted to open a small electronics item like a mouse knows that cutting through the plastic is no mean feat. I noticed ten minutes later that once it was removed from its oyster casing, the pulse oximeter was an attractive looking, curved, ergonomically designed, plastic alligator clip that measured an inch wide, two inches long, and an inch deep. I admired its "comfortable fingertip grip" and its "easy application," but I struggled with the meaning of one bullet point on the cover that stated, "Not made with natural rubber latex." I wondered why being made "with natural robber latex" was a bad quality. On the other hand, perhaps person #92-74031 who wrote that description of this "Made in China" instrument did not have a proper feel for the English language. A quick look at the instruction sheet, which was vaguer than an Ikea blueprint for assembling a bookshelf, confirmed the accuracy of my latter theory. I let the matter go without further reflection because I had a much larger task to accomplish.

My oximeter package included a lanyard, so I could carry it around my neck all day. Sonia expressed no interest in the oximeter, but she indicated that there was another, more elegant use for the lanyard. I studied a picture which demonstrated the "easy application" quality of the device and found that its Acme-simple claim appeared to be accurate. I would press together the hinged ends of the oximeter and insert my finger into the other end. Once my finger was inserted "nail side up into the maw until resistance is felt," the unit would "close gently below the first knuckle of the finger" so that sensors that I could not see would "align with the finger nail and pad at the tip of the finger (Fig. 1)." Figure 1 consisted of two figures, but I knew what the person was trying to say. Once my finger was in its proper position, all I had to do was press the power button (Fig. 2) and bingo-matic numbers would magically appear.

The suggestion that I would push a power button struck me as premature. I looked at the bottom of the third column of the instruction sheet and found the "Battery Installation and Replacement" clause. The gizmo was not going to work if I did not properly insert two AAA batteries, which the packager had kindly included with my oximeter. It was more difficult to open and close the battery compartment cover than I had anticipated, but I worked the problem, inserted the batteries properly, closed the cover, and touched the power button to see if it would light up or if the oximeter would explode.

I assumed it worked when it began flashing its own Morse code dashes and dots, so I skipped reading the "Troubleshooting" paragraph of the instruction sheet. Instead, I studied the "**IMPORTANT SAFEGUARDS**" section. "To avoid electric shock" I should take care "not to immerse the unit in water," nor should I "touch the unit with wet hands." Although I did not believe that a total charge of three volts would electrocute me, I did not want to wreck the inner workings of my oximeter before I got my first reading, so I took care not to drop it into Sonia's water bowl.

I realized that my procrastination and my obsessing over this tertiary information was caused by my fear of taking a reading and discovering that I would score in the mid to high sixties. I prayed that my score would be at least eighty. Such a high number would give me enough time to call a taxi for a quick ride to 251 E. Huron Street, where the ER doctors at Northwestern Memorial Hospital would know what to do with me to avoid my being vented. They must have read Dr. Levitan's study. I had printed a copy of it, which I would bring with me for quick reference, just in case they had no opportunity to peruse yesterday's New York Times.

Realizing that if I did not like my initial score I could re-test myself until my finger went numb or the two AAA batteries died, I braced myself and inserted my finger. Any finger except a thumb would do, but since the middle finger purportedly gave the most accurate score, I used that one. I rested my hand on my mouse pad and pushed the power button, feeling dizzily like I had inserted a voucher into a dollar slot machine at the Grand Victoria Casino and I was now waiting to see if three red sevens would appear.

I was elated to see the number ninety-seven appear upside down, less enamored when the ninety-seven changed to a ninety-six which morphed into a ninety-five. This was going the wrong way, I thought, and I considered stopping the test while I was still at ninety-five, as if I were playing a twisted version of Deal or No Deal and I could bank one hundred thousand dollars instead of risking it all for the grand prize of a million dollars.

The downward spiral continued "turning and turning in the widening gyre." My pulse increased as my oxygenation level decreased. Then suddenly, for some God only knows reason, my oxygenation level of eighty-nine changed to a ninety, and I beheld an awesome change—my level rose steadily, before it settled on ninety-six, where it remained for two minutes. I would have continued staring at the reading for an hour, but I wanted to conserve my batteries because I would be doing a great deal more testing, and because I was quite content with scoring a ninety-six.

My instruction sheet provided no guidance about what to think of readings that fluctuated so radically. I wondered if it was a typical trend, and if the device was functioning properly. I realized that re-testing throughout the day would provide a partial answer. When I received my Casper Oximeter courtesy of O'Bannon's Balms, I could compare scores. If both devices provided close to identical scores after x number of trials, I would conclude that the devices were reliable. If scores were widely disparate, well, I would need to purchase a third device, and onward from there until either the supply of oximeters in the world or my checking account was exhausted.

I shredded my instruction pages, written in five languages, all of which I assume were equally confusing. Sonia had grown tired of the lanyard, so I added it to a pile of some of her other toys. I put my non-natural rubber latex oximeter on top of my file cabinet, next to my framed lobby card from the film American Hot Wax. The oximeter would earn a permanent place of honor there if it continued to behave itself and supply me with the test results I wanted to see.

In each of the eight other times I re-tested myself that day, my score ranged between ninety-five and ninety-seven. When my second oximeter had arrived on Thursday of that week, I had charted similar scores in each of four daily finger insertions. The Casper Oximeter bore out those findings within one point on each test that day, and for the next two week that followed. It did not matter if I took the test before or after breathing exercises, before or after I did two hundred sit ups, or before or after eating. The results did not vary. Sometimes I reached an exhilarating pinnacle of ninety-eight; other times I bottomed out at ninety-three.

I was at a loss to figure out why, by the second week of May, I was coughing so frequently and why my headaches and loss of focus had not dissipated. My oxygenation levels were good. I followed my daily routine and I thought I was doing everything I could to feel better. I would have viewed the incongruity as another COVID-19 Mystery, but from what I saw on television and what I read online, I should have been feeling better by then. I was grateful that according to my twin oximeters I was not experiencing any form of hypoxia, but still, I felt oddly like Dave Bowman in <u>2001: A Space Odyssey</u> when Mission Control told him "this conclusion is based on results from our twin Niner-Triple-Zero computer." No matter what "cross-checking routines" were employed "to determine the reliability of this conclusion," Dave knew that something was wrong onboard The Discovery. I had undergone three failure-to-breathe-late-at-night episodes, and I had no confidence that I would not encounter a future one.

My personal Mission Control was the Illinois Department of Public Health. I was surprised to receive a follow-up phone call on May 14 from a different representative employed by that Department.

I remember the date because on May 14 the Supreme Court reversed Wisconsin Governor Tony Evers' decision to keep businesses closed and ordered him to "open immediately" restaurants and bars from Racine to Green Bay. Evers had not reached his decision lightly. He was guided by Dr. Fauci's testimony on May 12 when Dr. Fauci warned senators that re-opening too soon would result in "needless suffering and death."

At the behest of the Supreme Court, Chicagoans could now make the forty-minute drive to partake in Wisconsin Fever, joining fifty or sixty patrons hoisting a few New Glarus Spotted Cows on tap. Pleasantly inebriated, they could drive home to regale friends, relatives, and neighbors with tales of their exploits, inviting them to sign on to accompany them on their next foray into the Land of Sky-Blue Waters.

I was asked by my IDPH caseworker to verify my identity. After doing so I provided the rep with my first date of symptoms and my date of testing. The woman with whom I was speaking wanted to know what types of symptoms I had experienced. I ran down the list for her, but my descriptions were often interrupted by my coughing. She asked if my symptoms were gone. I assured her that, regretfully, my cough, headache, and loss of focus were still present. She asked if I was the only person at home and if I had any pets. I told her Sonia my cat was close by the entire time. The woman wanted to know if Sonia had displayed any COVID-19 symptoms, and I asked how those symptoms would be manifested in a cat. She said that vomiting blood would be a telltale sign. Relieved, I assured her that there had been no such indicator.

I was then asked to identify my race. After I told her Caucasian, she asked if I was a Health Care worker or a First Responder. She queried if I had received materials informing me how to protect others from COVID-19. I answered, "If you mean the pages of the Community Based Testing Site handouts, yes, I received them, memorized them, and told my friends about them." Satisfied with that reply, she asked if I had any recommendation for other COVID-19 patients.

I suggested three survival tips that I had found to be valid, reliable, and important. I told my case worker that driving should be avoided; that patients should get as much sleep as possible and not feel worried or guilty about doing so; and that having an oximeter or two on hand was crucial for monitoring lung functions.

She concluded her portion of the obligatory call by asking if I had any questions. Although I felt like I had been here before, I asked her why I had experienced breathing difficulty when my oxygenation level was normal; why I still had a cough, headaches, and loss of focus when it had been six weeks since I was tested; and how long should I continue to self-quarantine.

To my surprise and her credit, my IDPH representative did not default to the more typical "ask your medical practitioner" response. She asked me if I had documented my oxygenations when I experienced those late-night bouts of nonbreathing. I recognized where she was going when I told her "No, I did not own an oximeter at the time." She explained that oxygenation levels vary over weeks, and perhaps my level was not normal when I lost autonomous breathing capability for short periods of time. The concept made sense; perhaps if I had taken oxygenation readings during those frightening times, I would have been at mild to moderate hypoxia levels.

She asked if I had forgotten to mention a fever when I recounted my current symptoms. I replied that an elevated temperature was no longer a problem. She asked when my fever broke, and after I gave her that date, I told her I did not possess oximetry capability at the time. She informed me that "oxygen levels often improve when temperatures decrease." She said she was reporting observational data and that I should draw no conclusions.

I thought it helpful but unusual that she would have this sort of data on hand, and I asked her if she was describing incidental reports that she personally had heard, or if a formal database existed from which she was drawing her remarks. She said it was a combination of the two. I mentioned that I thought it would be helpful if COVID-19 patients in Illinois had access to that information. She said that the possibility was being investigated.

Regarding my coughing, she volunteered that although senior patients reported that an uncomfortable cough persisted for two to three months, in most cases the urge to cough eventually subsided. I pressed my luck and asked if the Coronavirus could have damaged my lungs permanently, but she said that I needed to "consult my doctor" for an answer to that question. I thanked her for her candor and when she ended the call, I added "get a referral for a chest x-ray" to my list of things to do.

The information I received from that call was unexpectedly reassuring. I would continue my routine for as long as it would take for my cough and headaches to abate. If that process took another month or so, I deemed the time spent a small price to pay to avoid death from COVID-19. Perhaps it would not take that long to recover. Either way, for the first time in months I could see a light at the end of the tunnel. It was more of a penlight than a klieg light, but it was a discernible sight with quantifiable properties.

The mystery that shrouded the Coronavirus mechanisms and the uncertainty about my ability to avoid its endgame had lessened. The disease still loomed as an inescapable, formidable, and threatening presence, but now I had the distinct and comforting feeling that I had somehow deflected the worst threats that the Coronavirus could throw my way, and within a relatively short timeframe, I would be healthy, and my need for self-quarantining will have ended.

I said a prayer of thanks. I played with Sonia. I embraced the rest of that day's routine with an air of optimism that had been a long time coming. I concluded that the dosage I received from The Sneeze was not large enough to kill me. I did not want to jinx myself; but I began to believe the cytokine storm had ended, and although no majestic rainbow appeared, I felt that there were considerably fewer clouds darkening my horizon.

One of the pratfalls of do it yourself COVID-19 survival is that at any time, under unforeseen circumstances, an action taken to prevent symptoms from worsening might have unintended and unwanted side effects. For example, although I had marginally raised the acidity of my bloodstream, I was no longer interested in waging a Manichean battle with COVID-19. I wanted a victory. I wanted to purge the Coronavirus from my system. I required a progressive circumscription of its evil intent until it gone and never would return, in the manner and with the same finality that Milton described Good conquering Evil in Paradise Lost. In my enthusiasm to recover I forgot that no single strategy could defeat the Coronavirus. I thought I could deliver a knock-out punch to the Coronavirus if I drastically increased the amount of grapefruit juice that I was drinking, making juice my go-to method of hydration instead of Gatorade and soda.

Two days later I found I could not move the front of my foot very adeptly. My big toe seemed frozen painfully in one position. The joint had reddened and was swollen. I found on WebMD that these were typical signs of gout, caused often by acidity in red wine or by juices with high acidity levels. Realizing the error of my way I halted all grapefruit juice consumption and removed Vitamin C and L-Arginine from my regimen for three days, which is how long it took for my toe and foot to stop throbbing and hurting. I reintroduced the vitamin and supplement gradually into the mix, but I shied away from drinking grapefruit juice in any quantity.

I was glad my recklessness and impatience had not caused me to develop gout. Prednisone was the recommended treatment for gout, and I saw online that "people taking oral corticosteroids (like prednisone) on a routine basis for such conditions as asthma, allergies, and arthritis may be unable to mount a normal stress response to the new coronavirus and are at high risk of doing poorly if they get COVID-19."[7] In other words, COVID-19 patients taking prednisone "experienced more severe disease once infected because these medications suppress their own steroid response to infection."[8] I hoped that my CIDP did not return until after a Coronavirus vaccine had been discovered, because both immunoglobulin and prednisone were no longer realistic means of therapy.

My black tea delivered more caffeine than my metabolism needed, and what did not bother me before now caused stomach distress. It may have also accounted for some of the tossing and turning I was doing throughout the night. I tested that theory by skipping black tea for two days and drinking thyme tea instead, but I still experienced mild insomnia and stomach distress.

Although my appetite had not returned, I followed my diet religiously. I did not skip a dinner no matter how ill-inclined I was to eat. I could not eat a great deal of food at any single sitting, so I tried to snack throughout the day and evening. I thought if I added more seasoning to foods, perhaps to a salmon steak that I had purchased from Costco which I kept frozen for six months, I would be inclined to eat more. Unfortunately, no matter which type or how much of seasoning I added to my salmon, it still tasted bland.

To be fair, the very thought of blackening a perfectly acceptable piece of salmon with a thick coating of lemon pepper, sage, and oregano was off-setting. Consequently, it came as little surprise to me when I climbed on my Hammacher Schlemmer Easy to Read Analgog Scale and saw that my weight had dropped to one hundred and sixty-five, down twenty pounds from the beginning of March. I had decided to cut down on desserts so that I would not become diabetic, but if this rate of decline continued, in a month I would become seriously underweight for a man of my age and height. Anyone who has tried to eat when not feeling hungry knows that you can ingest some food, but you did not want to spend three hours dining in the Bacchanal Buffet at Caesar's Palace. I decided that I would try watching a show like <u>Diners, Drive-Ins and Dives</u> on the Food Network an hour before dinnertime. Maybe the sight of Guy Fieri surveying a tall stack of loaded nachos would whet my appetite.

Disregarding those ephemeral inconveniences and given the undefined size of the Coronavirus dose I had received, I was confident that if I had not taken the measures I had employed, my symptoms would have been more severe, and my outcome might have been worse. Some of the actions I took to mitigate the effects of the Coronavirus had unintended and positive side effects.

By completing and updating lists of household chores, medications, meals, and safety measures, I created a discipline which I would find useful if my COVID-19 brain remained in stasis and affected my life in unanticipated ways. I would extend the use of lists to include work-related items, if selling airline tickets and generating hotel contracts regained viability as a future source of revenue.

Once I ruled out alcohol and cannabis as credible or effective Coronavirus therapies, I had no urge to partake in either for recreational purposes. I realized that abstinence from alcohol should be part of my future well-being once COVID-19 ceased to threaten my life. I recognized that avoiding alcohol would likely increase my life expectancy. I would use high CBD/low THC forms of edible cannabis to deal with arthritis and pain from injuries should those ills befall me. Regaining my previous yoga capabilities would also help me fight any debilitating disease while helping me attain better physical balance.

The weight I lost due to my lack of an appetite had significant and compound positive benefits. Maintaining a lower weight would reduce my chances of becoming diabetic or having a heart attack. Once my COVID-19 symptoms passed, a lower body/mass index was likely to reduce my blood pressure, which would eventually eliminate my need to take Lisinopril. Once I was able to exercise more often, my lower weight would also allow me to reduce my Atorvastatin dosage from eighty milligrams to half that amount. Given enough time and an encouraging blood screen, I might be able to forego the statin. If I continued to drink my Ninja Nuke and decaffeinated green tea each morning, I may no longer need to take Omeprazole.

In late May I realized that I should look at my wall calendar as part of a subset of daily chores. I was aware of the date of the month because I had kept a current log of my temperature, pulse, and oxygenation level. The tops of the compartments of my seven-day pill container were labeled AM and PM, which had become an important distinction, because in the worst of those dark, feverish days, I could easily confuse a gloomy morning for twilight.

It would have been helpful if I had specified days of the week in my notebook. Had I done so, I might have felt less banished within a grayish, timeless world of COVID-19, one in which I had become The Man in the Iron Mask, a prisoner marking the passing of each solitary day with a single line etched into the stone wall of my cell, using a sharp piece of rock I had pried loose from my cell floor as my primigenial marker.

I had slept fitfully each night as I awaited a reprieve from my dismal fate. Each waking hour I had searched the internet in vain, looking for new information about a Coronavirus cure. In doing so I had become the forlorn shipwreck victim on desert island who searched the skies for a rescue plane that would never arrive, praying for a sign from Above that help was on the way.

Occasionally an optimistic report would surface, distracting me temporarily from the horror of a rising death toll. By following rigid lockdown measures adopted by most countries in the world, the amount of carbon dioxide being pumped into our atmosphere had declined by seventeen percent in a two-month period. Resurrected or newly built drive-in theaters gained popularity. Restaurants specializing in all-you-can-eat buffets never re-opened. Shopping online became more widespread without a commensurate increase in online fraud. The National Basketball Association playoffs and Major League Baseball games began in July, both without live spectators.

The price of gasoline dropped to less than a dollar a gallon, which was a double-edged sword. The lower cost made essential trips more affordable for non-COVID-19 persons, but the drop in the price also encouraged people to travel more, which was not in anyone's best interest. Sales of huge recreational vehicles increased dramatically, allowing many cabin-feverish Americans to begin their sojourns to states that had not imposed COVID-19 travel restrictions. Alaska, Connecticut, Florida, Idaho, Illinois, Kansas, Maine, Massachusetts, New Hampshire, New Jersey, New Mexico, New York, Pennsylvania, Rhode Island, South Carolina, and Vermont were not accepting visitors in conveyances like the Winnebago Vectra and the Coachmen Sportscoach.

Because gasoline prices had dropped so radically, driving long distances in recreational vehicles at a rate of five or six highway miles per gallon became more affordable but not recommended, due to the extraordinary amounts of carbon emissions these vehicles pumped into the atmosphere in a weekend outing to the Wisconsin Dells. Tractor Town re-opened for a short while, which allowed professional landscapers, who did not wear masks, and desperate, amateur landscapers who did not wear masks to go forth with their seeding and multiply. Many of those practitioners spent weeks cultivating gardens while discussing politics with neighbors, none of whom wore masks.

The best national news by far occurred on July 23, when President Trump announced that he was cancelling the Jacksonville component of the Republican National Convention. Many elderly Republicans had informed the RNC that they would not attend, citing vague and spurious reasons like "schedule conflicts." To place the significance of their abstentions in its proper context, politicians live and breathe to attend a convention such as this one. It is what they do; it is their raison d'etre. On this occasion, however, party kingpins took a pass, believing it was important to miss the festivities so they might continue to live and breathe. I was glad the event was cancelled for any reason because countless lives were saved.

On the international front, self-isolated, elderly individuals found creative, often amusing ways to entertain themselves during the lockdown, and sometimes a humorous pattern of behavior would catch the eye of the world press. For example, premature violation of lockdowns had an unusual effect on the pensioner residents of Stevenston in Ayrshire, Scotland. They were concerned that due to lower petrol costs, a "lockdown at (Ardeer) beach was being flouted by a nudist influx."[9]

One resident focused on parking logistics, not naturism. He complained "They shouldn't be travelling from outside the area during lockdown. People turn up in cars, leave them outside our houses, then walk over."

Although their beach had "plenty of scope for nude walking," another resident who observed the nudity commented, "I can see them from my window. They have always got a backpack on. You wouldn't think it's good for germs." It was not clear if the resident objected more to the nudity, the backpack, or the germs. No slacker he, the resident committed himself to the onerous task of observing the textile-free parade each morning.

With binoculars in hand, he catalogued these migrations with painstaking precision. He did not record the position of the backpack on each of the four hundred and twenty-one naked bodies he spotted on an average day. He maintained his own social distance by standing on his porch and using the telephoto lens on his Canon A-1 camera to capture these damnable offenses to his sensibilities. The one hundred and two photographs he took provided all the evidence necessary to convict these ne'er-do-wells of ostentatious and invidious violations of lockdown protocol.

By the end of May, my coughing and headaches had ended. I continued to test my oxygenation level twice a day, to take my temperature every morning, and my blood pressure each evening. I was thankful for the prayers, kind words, and assistance of my friends and relatives.

On June 1 I ended my self-quarantine. I remained vigilant, and I exercised caution when venturing outdoors, because I did not know if I had developed an immunity to COVID-19. If I had an immunity, I did not know if my immunity was short-term, or if it was a "durable," that is, a long-lasting immunity. Perhaps I had developed what epidemiologists call "antibody dependent enhancement," where the number of antibodies in my system would not be sufficient to protect me from re-infection. I also did not know what a chest x-ray would reveal about the condition of my lungs, or if I would qualify for a monoclonal antibody test, which was another measure tightly controlled by the Illinois Department of Public Health.

I was aware that the world I was about to re-enter was in turmoil. In February, large cities were Coronavirus epicenters. Our major cities were still under its first-wave attack, but to make matters worse, cases of infection were spiking in rural areas in most states. Cities that had prematurely re-opened were forced to reengage lockdown protocols.

The challenge of surviving the Coronavirus pandemic had increased in its level of difficulty. Its spread was due, once more, to our usual suspect. By paying no mind to the uncontrolled spread of the Coronavirus, President Trump declared the pandemic irrelevant. It held no more sway over his actions than did the Constitution of the United States. Acting on his misbegotten belief that he could put the whammy on protestors by beating out of us our urge to exercise our right of free assembly, the President continued to wage his war of attrition on the lives and liberties of all Americans.

Chapter Six

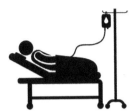

A Twice-Told Tale

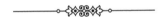

By April 1, every aspect of life in the United States had changed. Our jobs, our economy, our patterns of interaction with each other had been inexorably altered in ways that epidemiologists had predicted, and economists had feared. Hospitals ceased all elective surgeries. Essential procedures such as chemotherapy regimens were delayed until the risk of COVID-19 infection at hospitals had been reduced, and until ICU-bed and personnel capacities increased.

Traditional opportunities for employment had disappeared. Bars were closed and restaurants could offer only carry-out services. All sporting events were cancelled. The doors of chapels and churches were shuttered. Family gatherings at masses, weddings, and funerals ceased to exist. The few hotels that remained open operated at five percent of standard capacity. Air travel had stagnated. The TSA screened fewer passengers per day than at any other time in its nineteen-year history, that is, until July, when the number of domestic passengers dropped below the inauspicious record set in April.

We lived in the face of two fears: that we could be infected by the Novel Coronavirus on any given day, and if we were not infected this summer, infection and death could occur due to a second wave of COVID-19 in the fall. Those fears were as palpable as the fear of nuclear annihilation that we experienced during the Cuban Missile Crisis.

A few weeks after the Wuhan City fireworks celebration ended and the town, along with the rest of Hubei province, opened for business on April 8, after its seventy-six day shutdown, a resurgence of cases of COVID-19 was reported in Wuhan and in the city of Shulan in Jilin province. In response to that alarming development, the Chinese government ordered that all eleven million Wuhan City residents and the seven hundred thousand residents of Shulan be tested for COVID-19. Individuals who tested positively were quarantined. The strict quarantine made contact tracing feasible, because the number of persons contacted by a quarantined person was limited. The further spread of those outbreaks ended. Wet markets were permitted to re-open, but the government "stopped the sale and consumption of wild animals in response to the coronavirus."[1]

During that same timeframe, our federal government did *nothing* to increase the widespread testing of its citizens. In fact, every action our government took made it *more difficult* for states to conduct extensive testing. Governors who asked for more tests were told to fend for themselves. By the third week of July, all beds in hospitals in places like Hidalgo County, Texas were full. Incoming COVID-19 patients were put in reclining chairs in the hallways of hospitals located across the Rio Grande Valley. We had resorted to treating our COVID-19 patients with the same aplomb that characterized the treatment Wuhan City patients received when they were brought to warehouse at the beginning of the outbreak in January, where they were left to die in chairs because there was an insufficient number of hospital beds.

In neighboring Starr County, Texas, due to a lack of hospital beds and a critically low level of oxygen, health practitioners were forced to use pre-admittance screening to determine a patient's "survivability." Crisis care was previously defined by its utilization of a triage rating system, whereby only the sickest patients would be admitted for treatment. Now, when it appeared that a patient's symptoms were so severe that there was little chance he or she would recover if admitted to a hospital and if put on a ventilator, the patient was sent home to die.

Because there were so many dead COVID-19 victims, refrigerated trucks were brought onsite to store bodies for up to two weeks, until crematory space became available. This is the situation to which health care in the United States in 2020 had deteriorated, and it all could have been avoided if President Trump had implemented widespread testing throughout the country, in major cities, in rural areas, in counties like Starr County with one small hospital, in towns with meat processing facilities, in prisons, in areas of diverse ethnic populations, and in nursing homes.

On March 6 President Trump had declared that "Anybody that wants a test can get a test. That's what the bottom line is...Anybody right now and yesterday—anybody that needs a test gets a test. We—they're there. They have the tests. And the tests are beautiful. Anybody that needs a test gets a test."[2] The number of tests available to states was insufficient to test residents who wanted tests. Federal restrictions prohibited states from administering more than a pre-established quota of tests on any given day at any Community Based Testing Site. "Anybody" who had undergone a nasal swab test would concede that the experience was not beautiful.

The federal government blamed states for the inefficiencies and hardships we experienced. White House staffers referred to that plan as a "state authority handoff." Then on July 21, they further confounded plain-speaking Americans by describing the premature re-opening the economy and of public schools as a "mandate-easing scenario." Under that scenario, they predicted that six hundred and fifty thousand of us would die by the end of 2020. To make sure that his staffers would be able to adjust downward the actual number of hospitalizations and deaths that would occur by year-end, President Trump ordered that health care administrators send their data directly to his White House canaille, not to the Center for Disease Control and Prevention, which was the institution better equipped to collect, organize, and report on the number and trends of infections, hospitalizations, and deaths.

To minimize the significance of the ever-expanding number of positive cases and of COVID-19 deaths, President Trump stated the Coronavirus "will disappear," manifesting upon its exit the same flourish, grace, and ease of opportunity that Henry Hill displayed when escorting Karen Friedman into the Copacabana night club while the Crystals sang "Then He Kissed Me" in Martin Scorsese's 1990 film Goodfellas. Our total number of positive cases recorded on August 1 stood at four and a third million. That fact impelled President Trump to add, "I think we've really started it up very successfully." His statement was accurate if the ability to set record numbers of new infections and new deaths with each passing day defined President Trump's standard of success. From his lips to the ears of a hundred and fifty thousand bereaved families, his besotted words were the kiss of death.

The federal government pitted state against state in a struggle to procure tests. To make matters worse, our government engaged in bidding against states for the same tests, for the same N-95 masks, for the same protective gowns and shields. President Trump stated that this series of inappropriate, interconnected wrangling exemplified a "free marketplace" in action. Apparently, he was blissfully unaware of Adam Smith's notion that a free market meant a marketplace free from government interference.

Admiral Brett P. Giroir, our Assistant Secretary for Health and Human Services, often appeared at Task Force Briefings. Throughout April he meandered through the revolving door position of point man for the Task Force. Giroir was the person "in charge of testing." He took center stage during the April 27 briefing and announced an eight-part plan that governors would follow when re-opening their states.

Giroir thanked President Trump and Ambassador Burk, by whom he meant Dr. Deborah Birx, and then explained at light speed a plan so complicated that no one had a chance of understanding it. Using vague terms like "Emergency Use Authorizations," he proposed that we "Galvanize commercial and research laboratories." The eight-part plan soon encompassed eleven parts, because Dr. Birx's core elements of "Robust Diagnostic Testing," "Timely Monitoring Systems," and "Rapid Response Programs" needed to find a home within Giroir's scheme.

When he began his lecture, Giroir demonstrated he was unhappy using Birx's core elements to organize his plan, and so he divided his original octagon into three different parts. He called Points One to Five a **"LAUNCH;"** Points Six and Seven showed us a **"SCALE;"** and Point

Eight was categorized as "**SUPPORT OPENING UP AGAIN**." He chose to avoid common, everyday English phrases when talking about his generic "model." Instead he served us hogwash like "We had seventy-three of the two point oh sites going to one ten," which for him "demonstrated the model."

Trying to hide from his own confusion about what really should happen next, and confident that no listening to him had any clear notion of what he meant by his rambling disquisition on re-opening, Giroir stated that he would host another conference call with governors "to understand what their testing aspirations are." Everyone near the podium, in the Press Corps, and watching from home knew what the governors wanted. We could bet that, as far as the federal government was concerned, the needs and goals of blue state governors would forever and always remain as unfulfilled "testing aspirations."

I was amazed that Giroir could tell everyone without a hint of embarrassment that "the minimum that we're supplying to states is approximately double in that month than the Republic of Korea has performed." When he began his comparison, he said the double number referred to "supplies" that our governors would receive. At the end of Korea Calculation, he said the double number referred to "the amount of testing we're going to be doing." Either way, who really cares how we rate against South Korea? We do not pay our grocery bills in won. We are not relocating our households to Seoul in the foreseeable future. I wondered, if we allowed his outlandish comparison to stand, how Giroir would circumvent the fact that the number of tests performed in South Korea was instrumental in helping the country control its pandemic, while the "double" number of tests in this country had not made a dent in reducing our death toll.

I had to ask myself once more, "When will the stultifying talk end and the hard work begin?" The resounding answer was "never." When the Admiral stood before us in his dress blues, when he camouflaged the dire state of testing in our country by using inapplicable and phony statistics, I wanted to ask him "Do you feel like we do?" If I saw Giroir or his colleague Dr. Robert Redfield at the CDC on a street corner one day and asked either of them for a few dollars because I was out of work and I had not eaten in two days, both of them would explain to me for an hour using terms I could not understand why they were doing me a favor by not giving me ninety-nine cents for a Crispy Chicken Sandwich at Wendy's. I wondered if Doctors Giroir and Redfield had any notion of how betrayed we felt when they and their Boss fed us the same line of baloney day after day.

The Trump propaganda machine was formidable. It seemed that our two highest elected officials, President Donald Trump and Vice-President Mike Pence, and the political hacks who did their bidding preferred infinite rhetoric over finite actions. We accepted obscure phrases like "level of granularity" when it came from scientists like Dr. Brix and Dr. Fauci. We knew that was how they talked, and that at some point their meanings would be explained to us. Admiral Giroir, who was a doctor and should have known better, would not tamp down his overstated elaborations. He could be trusted to downplay the danger we faced. As a military man, he should have understood that death by lethal infection was a serious matter, since more soldiers died of disease in World War II than by battle injuries. Unscathed by facts, Giroir ended his time at the lectern by saying, "I'm very excited right now as we complete this ecosystem."

At what point in the Trump era, I wondered, had Newspeak replaced the English language? The ecosystem that concerned us involved the Coronavirus interacting with humans, and it was an ecosystem that we knew had not been completed. Admiral Giroir's misuse of language exemplified the relevance of Sam Spade's rebuke of Wilmer Cook's diction in The Maltese Falcon, when after listening to the hood's colorful threats, Spade replied, "The cheaper the crook, the gaudier the patter."

A similar accusation could not be leveled against President Trump. His repetition of simple adjectives such as "fake," "great," "sad," "beautiful," "amazing," "huge," "tremendous," "incredible," and "strong" in speeches and tweets, for example, is easily understood, but the usage demonstrates that his spoken and written vocabularies never progressed beyond a sixth-grade level. His reliance on name-calling, his use of pejorative nouns like "morons," "haters," and "maniacs," and his use of nonspecific phrases such as "a lot of," "good guys," "very bad people," and "total losers" illustrate the impoverished lexicon used more commonly by schoolyard bullies than by presidents of the United States. We were trapped in this whip-song, shackled between Admiral Giroir's feigned eloquence and President Trump's inarticulate utterances.

This specific press conference was not unique in its portrayal of style over substance, but it was a good demonstration of the White House's theory of the Re-Education of America. In the reign of Donald Trump, phony public officials with checkered pasts repeated in scandalously oblique terms what President Trump had stated in blatantly ignorant terms.

These "explanations" coming from public officials in whom we were supposed to place our trust were self-contradictory. Giroir championed the initialization of Emergency Use Authorizations, for example, as roadblocks when states pressed him for more tests and for technologies that would permit a quicker turn-around time when determining the results of those tests. Whenever Giroir wanted to put a positive spin on his Plan to Test the Country, he stated that he had issued an EUA for ventilators to be stockpiled or for tests to be amassed. The "EUA" term possessed the vagueness required for Giror to uphold or dispense with his own policies as he saw fit.

The use of these EUAs was an essential component in his plan to "revitalize" a national testing strategy that had never been vitalized in the first place. Giroir viewed an EUA as his "get out of jail free" card. When it suited him, Giroir regarded a standing EUA as irrelevant. For example, after President Trump declared that twenty-nine million doses of hydroxychloroquine should be distributed to states, Giroir ordered that wholesale distribution of the drug should not be impeded. President Trump did not want the untested hydroxychloroquine usage to be limited to hospitals. Hydroxychloroquine should be available, he thought, to anyone who wanted to use the chemical.

An Emergency Use Authorization limited the use of the drug to hospitalized patients. But because the President believed that hydroxychloroquine possessed the healing properties of snakeskin oil, Dr. Giroir peddled those wares, and in doing so willingly violated his oath to "Do No Harm." He told Stacy Amin, the Federal Drug Administration's chief counsel, that the FDA should approve sending the dangerous drug to independent retail outlets such as drug stores. In defense of that preposterous notion, Giroir wrote, "Needs to go to pharmacies as well. *The EUA matters not.* The drug is approved [and] therefore can be prescribed as per doctor's orders. That is a FINAL ANSWER."[3] His was not a GOOD ANSWER, but as far as our Admiral and our President were concerned, it was a good enough one.

Since Dr. Giroir had resolved the states' aspirational intentions of testing and since he had mapped out the interconnected nutrient cycles and energy flows of his Coronavirus ecosystem, the White House released a "Proposed State or Regional Gating Criteria." If a state wanted to "Advance to Go," it had to "satisfy" those "gating criteria." The guidelines to be met "Before Proceeding to Phased Comeback" were specific and robust.

Before entering Phase One of re-opening, in the subcategory of "**SYMPTOMS**," a state should show a "Downward trajectory of influenza-like illnesses (ILI) reported in a 14-day period, " and the state should have a "Downward trajectory of covid-like syndromic cases reported within a 14-day period" to match. In the "**CASES**" subcategory, states could move to Phase One only if they showed either a "Downward trajectory of documented cases within a 14-day period" or a "Downward trajectory of positive tests as a percent of total tests within a 14-day period (flat or increasing volume of tests)." Hospitals in states gearing up for Phase One had to "Treat all patients *without crisis care*" and were required to have a "testing program in place for at-risk healthcare workers, including emerging antibody testing."[4]

Further, each "core state" needed to possess these "**TESTING & CONTRACT TRACING**" capabilities:

- Ability to quickly set up safe and efficient screening and testing sites for symptomatic individuals and trace contacts of COVID+ results

- Ability to test Syndromic/ILI-indicated persons for COVID and trace contacts of COVID+ results

- Ensure sentinel surveillance sites are screening for asymptomatic cases and contacts for COVID+ results are traced (sites operate at locations that serve older individuals, lower-income Americans, racial minorities, and Native Americans)

Under the category of "**HEALTHCARE SYSTEM CAPACITY**," each state had to own these capabilities:

- Ability to quickly and independently supply sufficient Personal Protective Equipment and critical medical equipment to handle dramatic surge in need

- Ability to surge ICU capacity

The final requirements before moving to Phase One were called "**PLANS**." States were exhorted to:

- Protect the health and safety of workers in critical industries

- Protect the health and safety of those living and working in high-risk facilities (e.g., senior care facilities)

- Protect employees and users of mass transit

- Advise citizens regarding protocols for social distancing and face coverings

- Monitor conditions and immediately take steps to limit and mitigate any rebounds or outbreaks by restarting a phase or returning to an earlier phase, depending on severity

States that complied with all "gating criteria" included in this paperwork coming from the White House could move into Phase One. Remarkably, once a state was Phase One certified, its responsibilities, along with the responsibilities of the federal government, completely and irrevocably ended. Phase One, Phase Two, and Phase Three of the White House document *never mentioned* any additional requirement for state actions. If a state had *"no evidence of a rebound"* and therefore could *"satisfy the gating criteria a second time,"* they were in the clear, and they were immediately eligible to claim the Phase Two and Phase Three door prizes. No modes of proofs of meeting the gating criteria were established. If a state checked 'Yes" to whatever internal documentation they chose to proffer, they were in like Flynn.

All guideline in Phases One to Phase Three were directed at individuals and employers. The benefits of being rated a Phase Two individual were numerous. For example, individuals in Phase Two could return "to work or other environments where distancing is not practical." They were free to resume non-essential travel. For the most part, Phase Three could be described as the time when you close your eyes and pretend the Coronavirus pandemic never happened.

Employers too had a sweet deal when their state entered Phase One. A "Return to Work" order was allowed. Non-essential travel of employees should be minimized, but not forbidden. If they wanted to, they could consider providing "**SPECIAL ACCOMODATIONS**" for employees who might be part of a "**VULNERABLE POPULATION**." What the White House failed to realize or acknowledge is that the entire population of the United States is vulnerable to COVID-19 infection. The Coronavirus is an equal opportunity employer; it does not discriminate because of "race, color, religion, sex (including pregnancy, gender identity, and sexual orientation), national origin, age (40 or older), disability or genetic information." Though it is often thought to be a senior's disease, for example, it is not. Though the severity of its symptoms will vary depending on demographics, all of us, young and old, are equally capable of becoming infected and dying, or becoming asymptomatic transmitters of the disease.

The Gating Proposal was not elegant, but it was comprehensive, and it would have worked *if* there had been provision for enforcement. To say that these federal guidelines lacked teeth for citing infringements by states or employers would grossly understate the problem.

A simple addendum listing "**Penalties for Noncompliance**" would have done the trick. To view the problem from another angle, President Trump was quick to militarize our streets to quell peaceful protests. Why he was such a wimp about militarizing the nation in the fight against the pandemic is a question for the ages. Our Armed Forces would have responded positively and quickly to enforce measures that would save American lives. A pandemic curfew and national quarantine would have saved lives. It would have been costly to implement and to enforce a specific and targeted approach for containing the pandemic, but its cost would have been trivial when compared to the trillions of dollars that were squandered, misallocated, fraudulently used, or lost in a C.A.R.E.S. bureaucratic shuffle. If any part of our massive spending had worked, we would not have a higher national daily rate of infection in June, July, and August than we had experienced in March, April, or May.

No proscriptive measures for dealing with violations were outlined, and neither the CDC nor OSHA had authority to cite employers for failing to "adhere to federal guidelines." With a nod and a wink, Phases Two and Three permitted, some would say *encouraged* governors and employers to do whatever the hell they wanted to return their states or businesses to profitability.

The White House rhetoric rolled onward. Standards were set that were blanketly ignored when President Trump decided the time to re-open was now. Gateway criteria be damned, the governors were going to re-open, and yesterday was not soon enough. States were free to establish their own re-opening plans, which bore negative correlations to the federal gateway plan.

For example, Florida and Georgia possessed none of the required "**TESTING AND CONTRACT TRACING**" capabilities, but their beaches and hair salons were open prior to Memorial Day, no questions asked or answered. I know for a fact that no one at the Illinois Department of Public Health did any contract tracing when I tested positive for COVID-19. I am sure mine was not the only case in Illinois where no contact or surveillance tracing took place, and yet Illinois re-opened before it cleared the federal gateway hurdles. By May 20, fifty states were "in some phase of reopening,"[5] but none of them met the gateway criteria to enter Phase One. Three weeks later, Alaska, Arizona, Arkansas, California, Florida, Kentucky, New Mexico, North and South Carolina, Mississippi, Oregon, South Carolina, Tennessee, Texas, Utah, and Puerto Rico posted record high numbers of positive COVID-19 cases. Five weeks later, thirty-three states showed a daily rate of infections that was significantly higher than any previous daily average. On July 1, forty-five states showed geometrically sharp increases in positive cases, doubling their mid-June daily averages.

These spikes did not constitute a resurgence or a "second wave." Case numbers represented new highs on an ever-increasing continuum of a first go-round. Trump proponents, from his Cabinet members to his allies at <u>Fox News</u>, have argued that higher rates of infection are meaningless because more testing is occurring. Their conclusion is that the goal for increased testing in this country has already been met. Those sophists fail to point out two crucial facts.

First, our current makeshift, let-the-state-take-the-fall testing strategy puts us on par to test a million persons a month. It does not take a genius to figure out that at this rate, many of us will be dead and buried long before seventy percent of our population is tested. A University of Washington study concluded that "roughly 147,000 Americans could die from the virus by Aug. 4."[6] The study lowballed the figure, thinking social distancing measures would be in place throughout the summer to offset the spread of the pandemic. The UW model accurately predicted that four thousand, four hundred of North Carolina's residents would die. Many of those people opposed the re-opening of their state. Ten days after its Memorial Day parties ended, Texas saw a thirty-six percent increase in the number of positive cases diagnosed. It is likely that this tragic pattern of deaths from re-opening will be repeated forty-nine more times before August 4, 2020, when all states plus Puerto Rico update their Grim Reaper tallies.

Second, as the number of positive test cases rises, the death toll rises. More positive testing is decidedly *not* an opportunity for us to relax our efforts. No one should be offering kudos for a job well done at this stage of the pandemic.

To understand President Trump's dislike for evidence-based action and the dumb recklessness in his rush to re-open the states of the Union, it is helpful to recall a scene from the film My Cousin Vinny. During the pretrial arraignment, Judge Haller tells Vinny, "It appears to me that you want to skip the arraignment process, go directly to trial, skip that, and get a dismissal." Haller's logic encapsulates President Trump's plan for re-opening. Notwithstanding Dr. Fauci's insistent pleas to re-open in a safe and orderly manner, President Trump skipped the trial, defied authoritative and reputable scientific advice, and demanded that all states re-open, thereby proving himself right and everyone else wrong. He was not troubled by the tragically high price we would pay for his hubris.

Though states unilaterally lacked a history of declining numbers of symptoms, of positive cases, and of deaths, states re-opened and we suffered, once again, at the hands of our President's devil-may-care foolhardiness.

212

I watched in horror as a hundred thousand American died of COVID-19 from February to May, mindful that those deaths could have been avoided if our President had not played fast and loose with the facts. The story was repeated at the end of May, when the next hundred thousand deaths began to amass, courtesy of an arrogance that is President Trump's calling card.

President Trump's refusal to wear a mask in public in March and April 2020 gave many Americans tacit permission to violate one of the social distancing requirements that would reduce the spread of the Coronavirus. The result was a drastic increase in test-positive cases. In May and June, the same lesson was repeated, on larger scale. Because the President gave each state permission to enter Phases One, Two, and Three in violation of gateway criteria, they re-opened, and the number of test-positive cases multiplied.

A corresponding backlash resulted, worse than the anti-social-distancing, drive-by protests that had occurred months earlier in Annapolis. Individuals who wore masks were called Commies by others who believed the Coronavirus threat to our country was either a hoax or an aberration that had ended long ago.

Everyone in this country has the right to act stupidly, but no one has the right to endanger the lives and health of others by acting stupidly. To wit, the Universal Orlando Resort opened for business on June 7. Although I do not understand the need to visit a theme park in the middle of a pandemic, I do understand why Universal would want to get a leg up on Disneyworld, which set July 11 as its date for re-opening. Since non-essential travel is permitted in Phase One and Beyond states, Universal Resort attendees encountered tens of thousands of like-minded vacationers who flocked to Florida, a state with the highest rate of infections. I feel sorry for the Universal employees who are required to put their lives at risk so that little Joey from Asher's Fork, Kentucky can enjoy a ride on Hagrid's Magical Creatures Motorbike Adventure.

The philosophy of "our state is open so come to our theme parks, enjoy our water slides, attend unmasked political rallies, sing in the Phoenix church choir, and stay for the extended happy hour at PRYSM nightclub" defines the type of stupidity that puts us at risk. It would be terrible if everyone taking part in any of those risky outings rolled up in a corner and quietly died, in solitude, after their thirst to put their lives at risk in Florida and at the Wisconsin Dells and in Lake of the Ozarks, Missouri and in Tulsa, Oklahoma had been quenched. Unfortunately, they will not pass without taking several thousand unsuspecting friends or relatives or strangers with them. Such is the peril posed by skipping the careful trial-run, and rushing headfirst into Phases One, Two, and Three.

As is often the case when cogent scientific advice is ignored, President Trump's plan to re-open the economy backfired. Our economy suffered further devastation when new cases surged to seventy-three thousand, a record set on July 17, and new closure orders were initiated. Each time a city official tried to enact a shelter at home ordinance, a Republican governor would declare the prospective measure "moot."

Americans who base their actions on the selfish belief that the Coronavirus threat is over are culpable; those of us who understand the prevailing and inescapable seriousness of the Coronavirus threat and who act responsibly are heroes in our fight with this pandemic. Sure, we would all like to reacquaint ourselves with the warmth and camaraderie found on Oak Street Beach in June, with the wild Fourth of July familiarities found before final call at the Morrison Roadhouse, with the excitement of joining thirty-five thousand fans listening to "Eye in the Sky" before tip-off at a Bulls game in the United Center, but these are short-term pleasures that we are willing to forsake to offset the long-term and deadly threat posed by the Coronavirus. Children, and adults with childish mindsets do not understand the concept of delayed gratification. It is a psychology and a patience that we must master as a nation if we hope to limit the number of our citizens who will perish during this pandemic.

It is questionable if our economy could survive a lockdown that would last from one to two years. Nor can we hope for the hurly-burly of social life to resume tomorrow. Dr. Michael Osterholm, a former interim Director of the Center for Disease Control and Prevention, addressed the need for finding the middle ground, the one to which Dr. Fauci urged President Trump to adhere. Dr. Osterholm used the following analogy to explain the complexities at play when he stated, "I look at this with two guardrails. On one side is a guardrail where we are locked down for 18 months to try to get us all to a vaccine without anyone having to get infected or die. We will destroy not just the economy but society as we know it if we try to do that. The other guardrail is to just let it go and see what happens. We will see the kinds of deaths we just talked about and we will see healthcare systems that will literally implode. And so we've got to thread the rope through the needle in the middle."[7]

President Trump began the public relations campaign to minimize the fallout from the pandemic by assuring us in March that a maximum of two hundred thousand Americans would die from COVID-19. Dr. Osterholm crunched numbers in early June and offered this projection: "So it would not be unreasonable to say based on what I just shared with you with 100,000 deaths for 5% of the population infected, that somewhere between 800,000 and 1.6 million people could easily die from this over the course of the next 12 to 18 months if we don't have a successful vaccine." These frightening numbers flirted dangerously close to the minimum number of deaths that the White House predicted would occur under its "mandate-easing" scenario.

President Trump told the nation that we would win the war with the wraith that was the Coronavirus because the virus would magically disappear one day. This was the exact scenario that Dr. Osterholm found to be most frightening: "My worst-case scenario is that we see it suddenly start to disappear from this country right now. And people say what, how could that be worst case? That's the worst because if that happens, it means that it's not disappearing due to human behavior or anything we've put in place to reduce transmission. That would tell me that this is now acting like a flu virus even though it is a coronavirus. If it looks like a pandemic flu virus, then that would suggest that in late summer or early fall we could have a very significant wave of activity that would overwhelm society as we know it, healthcare wise and otherwise. That would be really a very unfortunate situation."

Sudden disappearance of the Coronavirus would be the President's dream come true because it would fulfill his prediction that it would disappear in the summer. On that front, the fantasy that President Trump upholds differs radically from Dr. Osterholm's scientific assessment: "My best scenario is that this just continues to burn on—it's with us, but it doesn't ever overtake us. We learn to live with the virus, and we are able to suppress it without destroying society as we know it. And we get a vaccine in 12 more months, and we're able to get that into people and it works effectively, at least for the short term." He believes "we're somewhere between those two. What we don't understand is exactly where yet."

Dr. Osterholm preferred the term "physical distancing" to "social distancing." When asked to expound on the difference, he asked, "Remember the choir participant who sang for two hours and transmitted the virus to 42 out of 60 people?" He explained that "exposure as a dose is a combination of time and amount." Dr. Osterholm believed that if a person does not wear a mask and is exposed to a dose, he or she could be infected in less than a minute. Wearing a mask would allow a person to be exposed to that same size dose for perhaps ten minutes without being infected. If a person never wore a mask in public, as is the practice of our Commander in Chief, it is a certainty that sooner or later, he or she will be infected by the Coronavirus. It is a fact and a logic that is inescapable, no matter how urgently President Trump and his supporters may wish it to be otherwise.

Pseudo-science espoused by radio and television talk show hosts supported the President's line of thinking. Dr. Phil claimed that car accidents and drownings in swimming pools created more deaths than the Coronavirus, forgetting that those two causes of death were not contagious. Dr. Drew Pinsky said an individual was more likely to be hit by an asteroid than to die of COVID-19, even though the odds of being killed by an asteroid are one point six million to one. At that rate, fewer than 200 Americans should have died from COVID-19. Dr. Mehmet Oz urged schools to re-open in August "even if it meant people would die."

The debate about re-opening schools centered on when they should open, not how safely they should open. The same bandied words used to explain why the economy had to re-open in a hurry were rehashed to insist that it was in everyone's benefit to open schools prematurely. Again, no lesson from past mistakes was heeded. For example, advocates of the dangerous and unsubstantiated use of hydroxychloroquine found a new proponent on July 27, 2020 in the person of Dr. Stella Immanuel, pastor of the Fire Power Ministries. She recorded a Youtube from the steps of the U.S. Supreme Court building in which she stated "Nobody needs to get sick. This virus has a cure—it is called hydroxychloroquine." Dr. Immanuel's previous claim to fame occurred in 2013, when she declared that witches and demons are the causes of debilitating diseases.

During the public assemblies that occurred throughout the nation following the tragic death of Mr. George Floyd, protestors wore masks for several hours. However, they were not constantly exposed to the Coronavirus for hours. Intermittent exposure would certainly have taken place during that timeframe, but unlike unmasked parishioners listening to an unmasked choir, protestors were outdoors, and they were in motion. Fox News opined that the protests were super-spreading events, but such claims were bogus. According to Fox, it was unsafe to protest, but perfectly safe to attend crowded, indoor political rallies in Tulsa and Phoenix.

The Fox argument was half-correct, in an unintended way. It truly was unsafe to protest. The source of immediate danger was an armed militia. President Trump called his agent provocateurs onto the scene to intimidate and to inflict bodily harm on anyone within clubbing distance. All military tools of the trade for quelling insurrection were present and utilized. Tear gas put lungs in jeopardy, rubber bullets that could maim and kill were fired, and President Trump declared with each passing, violent subjugation of peaceful protestors that he was victorious on the "battleground" that our streets and avenues had become. He threatened that actions of "left-wing rioters" would impel him to invoke the 1807 Insurrection Act and use the US Army to subjugate protestors. He buried the fact that protestors were not attempting to overthrow the government. He equated protesting with insurrection by publicly, repeatedly, and erroneously claiming that all protestors were looters, arsonists, and anarchists.

In truth, commanders of our armies, like Major General Christopher Donahue of the 82nd Airborne Division, wanted little do to with fighting Americans on American turf. They certainly would have agreed with the sentiments expressed in the 1998 Edward Zwick film The Siege, when Bruce Willis as General William Devereaux objected to the use of Armed Forces in New York City. Devereaux warned, "Trust me, senator, you do not want the Army in an American city. There is historically nothing more corrosive to the morale of a population than policing its own citizens. Which is why I urge you, *I implore you,* do not consider this as an option!" Had President Trump accepted advice such as Devereaux's at face value, he might not have ordered elements of military police and other unidentified factions of the Justice Department and the U.S. Marshall Service, outfitted as though walked off the set of Mortal Kombat, to go one-on-one with the good citizens of Washington, DC at Lafayette Park on June 1 at 630 p.m.

Though President Trump never instituted a national strategy for testing, he was quick to devise a plan for militarizing the nation. His actions seemed guided by the credo, "Act in haste, and let the American public suffer at leisure." For example, to help improve his polling numbers, President Trump needed to curry the favor of the Evangelical voter base. If a mounted police charge into peaceful crowd was required to clear his Bible-thumping way to St. John's Episcopal Church to appease those voters with a photo op, it was a small price for protestors to pay. He ordered a Protecting American Communities task force to deploy its unidentified federal troops in Portland, Oregon, for example, and to subdue peaceful protestors whom he said were committing acts of "violent mayhem." The troops randomly abducted and unlawfully detained protestors. When mothers of those young people gathered to form a Wall of Moms to protect their children, elite Border Patrol Tactical Teams used tear gas and flash-bang grenades to tear down that wall.

What President Trump does not understand about America could fill volumes, but one crucial item he could not fathom is that "capitulate" is not in our vocabulary. Americans are made of sterner stuff. We never have and never will be deterred by strong-armed tactics. Every component of our history indicates that we will resist oppression by exercising our Constitutional rights. Under the reign of President Trump, America may "no longer be the land of the free, but it is still the home of the brave."[8]

God only knows what mayhem will ensue when President Trump attempts to win the 2020 election by hook or crook. Multiple strategies are already in play, involving the systemic disenfranchisement of African-American voters; the elimination of mail-in ballots, even though mailing-in is Mr. Trump's and Kayleigh McEnany's method of voting; and the enforcement of "exact match" laws. I would not be surprised to see literacy tests and grandfather clauses used to suppress voters in November 2020, and there is no predicting what degree of covert international involvement will plague our election process. Any attempt to reform voting processes in states should have started in May 2020, but it did not.

The mechanisms that President Trump has assembled to win a second term are formidable. When contemplating "1983," Jimi Hendrix sang, "The machine that we built will never save us." It is a statistical certainty that the political machine Donald Trump is building will never save us from COVID-19.

If he does get re-elected, let's hope he has the decency to apologize to us and to promise to live up to a campaign slogan which should have been "I'll make it up to you next time around."[9] More likely is that he will try to convince us that the road to Shambala is paved with lies and cons, with more split-tongued devils doing his bidding. I wish Hunter S. Thompson would have been alive to provide his take on the President's handling of the pandemic. I am sure he would have expressed—with far more eloquence than I can garner—his outrage over a series of selfish, political atrocities so obscene "that its intensity would shame the gamekeeper in Lady Chatterley's Lover."[10]

Of Richard M. Nixon, Dr. Thompson wrote, "We will not see another one like him for quite a while. He was dishonest to a fault, the truth was not in him." If Hunter Thompson were alive, perhaps he would have seen in Donald J. Trump the likes of Nixon. He would have raised a stringent voice warning us of dangers we would soon face. Maybe one more voice would have been enough to defeat Donald Trump in his quest for the Presidency. Perhaps the memory of Hunter Thompson's words two generations later will inform our decision when we cast our ballots on November 3, 2020.

Fifty years after George Harrison referenced Richard Nixon in "Beware of darkness," when he sang "Watch out now, take care, beware of greedy leaders/They take you where you should not go," we find ourselves at another crossroads, at the mercy of our leader who, with every step down his greedy path, leads us into quicksand. Although he did not create the Coronavirus pandemic, he sure as hell is making it easy for COVID-19 to kill us. Our fears and frustrations re-emerge, with the intensity of a head-banging-against-a-wall migraine, when we realize that an anthropomorphized Coronavirus could have no stauncher ally in the United States than President Trump. He calls real news about the Coronavirus "fake" and creates invidious mythologies about the virus as though he were a Fluxus artist, adjusting reality to suit his egomaniacal whimsy.

President Trump's premature opening of the country echoes the pattern of willful neglect that characterized his February 27 dismissal of the

Coronavirus threat. Four months later, he repeated that sentiment, stating "I think it will disappear." The recognition that we are once more suffering at the behest of his personal and political megrims produces a frustrating, painful, and maddening feeling of déjà vu.

His excoriatingly stupid answer to the COVID-19 puzzle is to pretend we will collectively step into Mr. Peabody's Way-Back Machine and return to the blissful time before the things went south in Wuhan City. After all, like Youngblood Priest in Super Fly, President Trump was just "tryin' to get over." Unlike Priest, he lacked intelligence, street smarts, and a moral code.

Americans though were not getting over. By July 1, our Coronavirus pandemic was uncontrollable in most of our states. Governors who realized too late that re-opening had been a major mistake began to institute lockdown procedures. The ugly scenario that was unfolding before our eyes was one that we had seen before. People waited in lines for days to get a test. EMTs needed more time to bring critically ill patients into hospitals after they arrived by ambulance. Emergency Department doctors and nurses needed more time perform a rudimentary triage. Contract tracing was an impossibility because people who tested positively were not forced to quarantine themselves. The honor system of self-quarantining fell apart when the states re-opened and the rate of transmission increased.

When intensive care units were overwhelmed, out-sourcing began, and hospital systems were forced to employ a "crisis standard of care." This extreme protocol was a gateway criterion—if crisis standards were in place, a state *could not* enter Phase One. A crisis standard of care means that whenever a sick person, someone who may or may not have tested positively for COVID-19 was brought to a hospital for emergency treatment, his or her symptoms would be ranked on a scale, and only the persons who scored highest would be admitted. Unlucky individuals whose symptoms did not score high enough for them to deserve a bed were told to take two aspirins and do not call in the morning. Once more the pandemic response found in our cities towns and villages edged closer to the standards of care found in Wuhan City's warehouses of death, thanks to the callous indifference of President Trump.

For my part, as I cautiously re-entered the world in June 2020, the over-whelming sensation I felt was gratitude. I was grateful that God had spared me from death by Coronavirus.

I have continued preparing and drinking my Ninja Nuke. My morning and evening intake of vitamins and minerals has not changed. It will be a while before I feel like eating pasta again, and although my appetite never returned to its pre-COVID-19 state, I managed to gain a few pounds and am comfortable with a weight of one hundred and seventy.

I have been sleeping better, and now that I am cough-free, I could extend the time I devote to practicing guitar. Along with "Cold Jordan," I like to play Mondo Cozmo's "Shine." Because I was grateful to Axl Rose for taking Steve Mnuchin to task, I am learning Slash's guitar solos on "Paradise City."

The only time I touch alcohol is when I disinfect the countertops, door-knobs, or the steering wheel of my car with Clorox wipes. I also use the hand sanitizers that grocery stores kindly provide when I enter and exit those establishments.

Whenever I go shopping, I wear my N-95 mask. It is a little a hard to breathe after a long time; for example, it became uncomfortable after four hours of waiting in Costco for the tire serviceman to install my four new Michelin tires, which went on sale in June. To solve that problem, I walked to the far end of the parking lot where no customers were located. Halfway between the store and the Costco gas station, I removed my mask for twenty minutes. The fresh air was exhilarating. It was difficult to believe that I was standing outside and that I was not coughing, and I am glad that it will be a while before that feeling of relief subsides.

I wonder how my clients will feel about wearing a mask in airports and on airplanes for extended periods of time. Face coverings will be required for years, I suppose, until a workable vaccine is available, and the entire pop-ulation of Earth is vaccinated. Personally, I would not be able to endure wearing a face mask for the fourteen hours it takes to fly to Tokyo, plus a minimum of two hours in the airport prior to the flight and the two hours it takes to de-plane and pass through Japan customs and immigra-tion. Regarding shorter domestic flights, United Airlines announced that beginning on October 1, when emergency federal funding to airlines ends, thirty-six thousand employees would lose their jobs, while American Airlines estimated its job loss total to be twenty-five thousand. Routes and the number of planes servicing the remaining routes would be downsized.

Fortunately, I have no need or desire to fly anywhere. But I wonder how people will eat and drink on their flights while wearing a mask; how sanitary the bathrooms will be on any flights, foreign or domestic; if children will be policed to make sure they are wearing masks at all times; if the person sitting in a middle seat will sneeze and transmit the disease to everyone sitting adjacently or within twelve feet of the sneeze; if the pilots and the cockpit crew will wear masks the entire time, and if so, how clearly will they be able to communicate with air traffic controllers; and finally, how scary will it be to see flight attendants in blue PPE patrolling the aisles. That image brought me back with striking clarity to my memory of PPE-gowned Army workers at the Irving Park Community Testing Site. Etihad and other international airlines have required its flight attendants to wear hazmat suits during all flights, which was a thought that reminded me of Doctors Stone and Hall wandering through the streets of Piedmont, Arizona, searching for survivors while dressed in their BSL-4 survival gear.

Once arriving at their various destinations, I wonder how my clients will tackle the problem of finding acceptable hotel accommodations. Hotels that have not gone out of business are operating at one of two extremes. Some hotels will do nothing to scare guests, providing them with a bare minimum of changes required to accommodate everyone in this new Coronavirus world. Other hotels and hotel chains have opted for taking the temperatures of guests when they arrive, making sure the guests soak their hands in a gallon of sanitizers before being allowed to enter keyless rooms or suites and removing "high-touch" features like television remotes. Some hotels have imposed a cleaning surcharge if a guest decides to take a shower. As a travel professional, I do not intend to stay at a hotel until I have been vaccinated against every possible mutant strain of the Coronavirus.

Regarding cruise ships, I believe that it will eventually be safe to cruise Europe or the Panama Canal or Southeast Asia, but I do not foresee that eventuality occurring in 2020. If I go on a cruise it will be at least two years from now, and I will avoid massive crowds on middling lines like NCL and opt for the smaller, luxurious ships of the Windstar or Crystal Cruise lines. I would exercise the same caution when deciding on a land-based trip. Whether I visited an all-inclusive vacation resort in the Riviera Maya region of Mexico or one of the Sandals resorts in St. Lucia, I would not partake until I was vaccinated. From a business perspective I wish I held a different, more optimistic opinion, but such is not the case.

At some point in the future, I plan to get a tan at Oak Street Beach, but I will wait at least until the summer of 2021. I hope it will be safe by then to plop down my towel six feet from anyone else on the beach. If there is an Air Show in Chicago in the summer of 2021, I will be the person watching the event at home, on television. Between now and then, I will not be visiting my friends at the Countryside Bar.

Having come close to dying, I can no longer watch films ending with the protagonist's death. I would rather watch a trashy movie like John Wick: Chapter 3—Parabellum where against all odds the hero survives a non-stop series of lethal obstacles than see Ken Miles die at the end of a good film like Ford vs. Ferrari.

I have continued doing my breathing exercises, and even though my oxygenation number is stable at ninety-six, I will have a chest x-ray performed as soon as it looks safe to return to a hospital without contracting COVID-19. My absent-mindedness has dissipated, thankfully. My yoga poses and consequently my balance has improved.

I added running to my exercise regimen and eke out a slow four miles each morning. I thank God that I can put in the miles at any speed. To conserve the cartilage in my knees, back, and hips, I make each footfall as light as possible. I imagine myself floating above the surface; it was a technique I had observed when I watched Chariots of Fire. I admired how world class athletes Eric Liddell and Harold Abraham ran when they won their Olympic gold medals. There have been many great films about running, from The Loneliness of the Long-Distance Runner to McFarland, USA, but Chariots of Fire appealed to me the most because of the close identification Liddel made between succeeding at races and worshipping God. I am using the LSD-method of training, running long, slow distances to improve conditioning. I hope to run another marathon before I die.

I would like to spend fifteen minutes talking to President Trump. I would respect the Office, but I would not coddle the President's eccentricities. I would urge him to admit that at some point in these unholy times he had tested positive for COVID-19, and his miserable actions and regrettable omissions were the result of his diminished capacity. Now that he was feeling better, I would ask him to tell the nation that he would correct his missteps, that he would enact a national testing strategy, that he would empower the CDC to take the lead in controlling the pandemic using whatever means its directors deemed necessary, that he would respect the rights of peaceful protestors, and that he was deeply and sincerely sorry for all the injuries and deaths that his negligence had caused. I would assure him that if he followed that course of action, Americans would forgive him. Whether or not we would re-elect him in November was uncertain, but by doing what was right, his place in history would be assured.

One day when I was running on the bicycle path through the Forest Preserve, I spotted a doe and her two babies. As they stared at me, I was overcome by an understanding of their innocence. It had been so long since I had seen evidence of life unaffected by the Coronavirus that I nearly cried.

Sonia continues to do well. I reduced her dose of decongestant to one-half a milliliter administered every other evening, and she has been sleeping soundly and snoring contentedly. I hope the therapy will allow her to lead a long life free from pain.

If I knew I had acquired immunity to COVID-19, I would have joined the ranks of protestors in Chicago after the death of George Floyd. I watched them from my balcony as they walked three miles from Jefferson Park to Park Ridge on Northwest Highway. The sight reminded me of heady times forty years ago, when my friends and I stood in front of the Illini Union protesting the bombing of Cambodia during our sophomore year at the University of Illinois in Champaign. I recall standing a few yards from armed National Guardsmen, just as Washington, DC protestors faced military police at Lafayette Park.

On July 1, 2020, fifty thousand new COVID-19 cases were reported in the United States *in one day*. Instead of acknowledging that watershed moment, President Trump asserted, "People will be very happy with unemployment benefits." I applied for unemployment compensation in May. Three weeks later, the Illinois Department of Employment Security responded that I had earned no wages in the last three years. I filed an appeal in writing, asking why I had been paying state and federal income tax all those years if I had not earned any wages. I included a year of pay stubs. Another three months have passed, and I am awaiting a response. By adding an automatic disconnect function to its 800-244-5631 number, IDES successfully reduced the number of annoying calls it was receiving from more than a million unemployed workers who wondered why they were getting the royal run-around. None of those applicants are "very happy."

When the national count had reached fifty-five thousand new cases on July 2, I was reminded of a line from a song by Flogging Molly, when Dave King sang, "It's been the worst day since yesterday."[11] On the evening of the Third of July, the quality of our fireworks display on Mt. Rushmore far surpassed the quality of Wuhan City's re-opening celebration. Ours featured yet another annoyingly long-winded, rambling, racist speech by President Trump, who made political hay while the fireworks shined.

It is impossible to assess accurately the degree to which the Mt. Rushmore celebration precipitated the increase in the number of positive COVID-19 cases reported in Rapid City two weeks later, but common sense dictated that the prudent course of action would have been to follow the example set by Chicago when the city decided on July 2 not to host its traditional Navy Pier Independence Day celebration. Chicago's Mayor Lori Lightfoot did not give a Fourth of July speech at Navy Pier. Instead, she issued an Emergency Travel Order mandating fourteen-day quarantines for passengers arriving at Midway and O'Hare Airports from any states with high Coronavirus infection numbers.

The quarantine order affected many Illinois residents flying home from the South Dakota, where fifty-nine of the state's sixty-six counties, including Rapid City's Pennington County, posted new highs in Coronavirus infections. Washington, DC's Mayor Muriel Bowser cancelled firework celebrations in her city. Like a petulant child, President Trump countered by urging residents to gather in large crowds to attend airshows and fireworks displays, hosted by the White House. Two weeks later, the number of daily positive cases reported in our country exceeded seventy-three thousand.

We previously encountered a similar rate of increased transmissions two weeks after Memorial Day, but that lesson was lost on everyone who chose to gather in small and large groups not wearing masks to light M-80s or to ooh and ahh as massive shells, some weighing the same as my Toyota Corolla, illuminated the skies of Washington, DC. Once more, after the President demonstrated that it was time to party hearty, many Americans were willing to oblige. They experienced the best, and what very well could be the last Fourth of July fireworks display that they would witness.

My struggle to survive COVID-19 changed my life in three significant ways. I felt a renewed sense of spirituality. I had a deeper respect for all forms of life, except for the Coronavirus. I came to understand that anything is possible if I retain hope for a better future.

I also learned a few significant lessons in the months that it took for my illness to run its course. I summarized those recognitions by proposing to myself this series of hypotheticals.

If the battery of my Corolla had died on the morning of March 31 while I was waiting in line to receive my Community-Based Coronavirus Test, the last person on earth from whom I would seek help would be Donald Trump. I fear he would have trouble distinguishing between positive and negative cables and posts. For example, on May 21, when he attempted to tell the White House Press Corps that he did not have COVID-19, he gabbled until he finally came out with "I tested positively toward negative."

If I were in desperate need of having a prescription filled, the last person I would send to CVS would be Donald Trump. I fear that he would tell the pharmacist I needed some version of "a drug called chloroquine—and some people would add to it 'hydroxy.' Hydroxychloroquine? So chloroquine or hydroxychloroquine." Garrulous uncertainty over important details and his penchant for confusing names, dates, and previous statements he made works contrary to the "aura of legitimacy" President Trump believes he projects.[12]

If I were in a skyscraper and a fire broke out, the last person I would trust to pull a fire alarm would be Donald Trump. I would be afraid that, like the Defense Production Act, he would talk about how effective fire alarms were in directing firemen to go to where they were needed, but he would never activate the device and the building would burn, with me in it.

If I had to develop a new strategy to defeat an opponent in chess, the last person I would call for a consult would be Donald Trump. As was the case with our nonexistent National Testing Strategy, he would tell me that he had developed a beautiful plan, one which would work perfectly. When I sked, "But what is the plan, Donald?" he would proudly reveal that fifty other people plus one in Puerto Rico would solve the problem for me.

If I had searched in vain on the eve of the Fourth of July for one of Holly Fiegerman's sold-out, portable air conditioners because my central air unit had broken, even though I knew Donald Trump had ten thousand of the air conditioners stored in one of the ninety-eight empty floors of Trump Tower Chicago, he would be the last person in the world from whom I would ask for one. I knew that a month after he told me that anyone who needed an air conditioner would get one, I would be sweltering in the heat and humidity of August in Chicago, because not a single air conditioner would leave his stockpile.

Donald Trump would be my go-to guy if I sought instructions on how to run several businesses into the ground, how to declare bankruptcy, and how *not* pay workers the wages justly due to them. He would be number one on my speed dial if I wanted to wreck an economy and willfully neglect the needs of three hundred and thirty million people. If I needed a blueprint on how to lead the world in the number of cases of COVID-19 and in the number of deaths resulting from that disease, he would be the knowledgeable civil servant I would call.

The one thing that is certain in this life is that President Trump is not a good loser. If he falls far enough behind in polling, it is possible he will pick up his marbles and go home. If he loses the election by a large margin, I am certain he will display the same cordial graciousness toward the winner that Isiah Thomas and the Detroit Pistons offered to Michael Jordan and the Chicago Bulls after the Pistons lost Game Four of the 1991

NBA Eastern Conference Playoffs. If he loses by a small margin, he might declare the result "fake" and refuse to vacate the West Wing.

Whenever I see the endless stream of self-congratulatory hype, as Presidential press conference and rallies cascade into one another, I am acutely aware that too many Americans have suffered unnecessarily at his hand. When I look into President Trump's squinty eyes, I see nothing. No compassion. No remorse. No guilt. I see a mile-long stare. Perhaps there is a glint of condescension; I can no longer tell for sure. He certainly views us with detachment and disdain, two qualities that no American president should exhibit. His vacant words are manifestations of the lies he tells himself and repeats to us. In my nights of tossing and turning in COVID-19 fever, hoping for the temporary relief that sleep would bring, I wondered how America could have fallen prey to such a villain. Our only recourse is to work together to survive a few more months until November Third, when we raise a strong, proud, and courageous voice, proclaiming in unison that there will be a changing of the guard. Until that time, we must remember to "help each other, and be prepared for anything," because our war to survive the Coronavirus in the reign of Trump "has just begun."[13]

About the Author

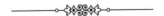

Gerry Plecki received his Ph.D. from the University of Illinois at Urbana-Champaign in 1979 and was awarded an NEH Post-Doctoral Fellowship at New York University. He has written articles on music and film criticism. His previous books were <u>Robert Altman</u>, which was an authoritative analysis of the director's films, and <u>Singing in the Rain: The Definitive Story of Woodstock at Fifty</u>, which was published in July 2019. He serves as Corresponding Secretary for the Society of Midland Authors.

Gerry gratefully acknowledges the words and opinions of the doctors, scientists, authors, singers, and songwriters cited herein. Their sentiments were a valuable source of consolation and inspiration.

Endnotes

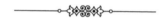

Chapter One

1   Hjelmgaard, Kim. "WHO says coronavirus came from an animal and was not made in a lab." <u>USA Today</u>, April 21, 2020.

2   Guzman, Joseph. "Experts: 90 percent of US corona virus deaths..." <u>The Hill. Com</u>, April 16, 2020, https://thehill.com/changing-america/well-being/prevention-cures/493128-90-percent-of-coronavirus-deaths-may-have-been

3   Haberman, Maggie. "Trade Advisor Warned White House in January of Risks of a Pandemic." <u>The New York Times</u>, April 6, 2020.

4   Miller, Greg and Nakashima,Eillene "President's intelligence briefing book repeatedly cited virus threat." <u>The Washington Post</u>, April 27, 2020.

5   Riechmann, Deb. "Sleuths at National Center for Medical Intelligence at Fort Detrick in Maryland tracked, warned of the new coronavirus." <u>The Baltimore Sun</u>, April 16, 2020, http://www.baltimoresun.com/coronavirus/bs-md-coronavirus-medical-intelligence-fort-detrick-20200416-snd2ky66rvdtbfr7mpj2ry-ofpe-story.html

6   MyNorthwest Staff. "Coronavirus deaths in Washington now up to 18, with 136 total cases." MyNorthwest, April 16, 2020, https://mynorthwest.com/1744551/live-updates-coronavirus-washington-state-2/?

Chapter Two

1   Eder, Steve et al. "430,000 People Have Traveled from China to U.S. Since Coronavirus Surfaced." The New York Times, April 15, 2020.

2   Dearen, Jason and Stobbe, Mike. "Trump administration buries detailed CDC advice on reopening." AP News, May 7, 2020, ttps://apnews.com/7a00d5fba3249e573d2ead4bd323a4d4

3   Sfondeles, Tina and Wittich, Jake. "Pritzker orders all bars and restaurants to close to dine-in customers by end of day Monday." Chicago Sun Times, March 15,2020.

Chapter Three

1   Ngan, Mandel. "China's Coronavirus Lies Don't Excuse Trump's Egregious Failures." CCN.com, April 2, 2020.

2   Hart, Melanie and Fuchs, Michael. "Trump's Coronavirus Survival Strategy: Blame China." Center for American Progress, April 14, 2020, https://www.americanprogress.org/issues/security/news/2020/04/14/483119/trumps-coronavirus-survival-strategy-blame-china/

3   Parker, Mario and House, Bill. "Trump's GOP Blames China for Coronavirus With Eye on 2020." Bloomberg.com, April 15, 2020, https://www.bloomberg.com/news/articles/2020-04-15/trump-s-gop-blames-china-for-coronavirus-with-eye-on-2020-races

4   Chait, Jonathan. "Trump Campaign's Genius Plan to Blame China for the Coronavirus Has One Flaw." NY Mag's The Intelligencer, April 14, 2020, https://nymag.com/intelligencer/2020/04/trump-china-biden-coronavirus-false-travel-ban-wuhan.html

5   Chait, Jonathan. Trump Campaign's Genius Plan to Blame China for the Coronavirus Has One Flaw." NY Mag's Intelligencer, April 14, 2020.

6   Dorman, Sam. "Sen. Murphy says Trump, not China or WHO, to blame for US coronavirus crisis." Fox News Channel, April 15, 2020, https://www.foxnews.com/media/chris-murphy-trump-to-blame-coronavirus-crisis

7   Smith, David. "Trump fans flames of Chinese lab corona-
    virus theory during daily briefing." The Guardian, April 15,
    2020, https://www.theguardian.com/world/2020/apr/15/
    trump-us-coronavirus-theory-china

8   Porter, Tom. "Trumps says China..." Business Insider,
    April 19, 2020, https://www.businessinsider.com/
    trump-says-china-may-have-started-coronavirus-deliberately-2020-4

9   Detsch, Jack and Gramer, Robbie. "The Coronavirus Could
    Upend Trump's China Trade Deal." ForeignPolicy.com,
    April 21, 2020, https://foreignpolicy.com/2020/04/21/
    coronavirus-trump-china-trade-war/

10 Burns, Robert et al. "Iran-US tensions rise on Trump
    threat, Iran satellite launch." ABC News, April 22,
    2020, https://abcnews.go.com/Politics/wireStory/
    trump-tweets-ordered-navy-destroy-iranian-gunboats-70284516

11 Burns, Robert et al.

12 Kelleher, Suzanne Rowan. "Photos: Florida Governor Opens
    Beaches, Crowds Appear Immediately." Forbes.com, April 18, 2020,
    https://www.forbes.com/sites/suzannerowankelleher/2020/04/18/
    photos-florida-governor-opens-beaches-crowds-appear-immediate-
    ly/#1779c493d183

13 Messer, Olivia. "Texans Brace for a COVID-19 'Explosion' Just
    Days After Reopening." The Daily Beast, May 5, 2020, https://
    www.thedailybeast.com/texans-brace-for-a-covid-19-explosion-just-
    days-after-reopening?ref=scroll

14 Mikkelson, David. "Did Texas' Lt. Gov. Say 'There Are More
    Important Things Than Living'?" Snopes, April 22, 2020, https://
    www.snopes.com/fact-check/patrick-more-important-living/

15 Messer, Olivia. "Texans Brace for a COVID-19 'Explosion' Just
    Days After Reopening."

16 King, Laura. "Governors shrug off Trump's insults as they
    plead for federal aid." Los Angeles Times, March 29, 2020,

https://www.latimes.com/politics/story/2020-03-29/
trump-governors-coronavirus

17 Bennett, John T. "Trump accuses Democratic governors of
    'mutiny' as he ignores constitution." Independent, April 14,
    2020, https://www.independent.co.uk/news/world/americas/
    us-politics/trump-coronavirus-constitution-democratic-gover-
    nors-a9464776.html

18 Rosen, Christopher. "Jimmy Kimmel Left Aghast by
    "Dangerously Misguided" Las Vegas Mayor." Vanity Fair, April
    23,2020, https://www.vanityfair.com/hollywood/2020/04/
    jimmy-kimmel-las-vegas-mayor-anderson-cooper

19 Liptak, Kevin. "Trump emerges from White House bubble to visit
    Arizona mask-making company." CNN.com, May 5, 2020, https://
    www.cnn.com/2020/05/05/politics/donald-trump-arizona-honey-
    well-white-house/index.html

20 Liptak, Kevin. "Trump emerges from White House bubble to visit
    Arizona mask-making company."

21 Capaccio, Tony. "US has gunships ready to deliver on Trump's
    warning to Iran." Stars and Stripes, April 25, 2020, https://www.
    stripes.com/news/middle-east/us-has-gunships-ready-to-deliver-on-
    trump-s-warning-to-iran-1.627376

22 Rupar, Aaron. "Why Trump's efforts to blame Obama for the coro-
    navirus make absolutely no sense." Vox, April 20,2020, https://www.
    vox.com/2020/4/20/21227903/trump-blames-obama-coronavirus

23 Heisler, Todd. "Models Project Sharp Rise in Deaths as States
    Reopen." The New York Times, May 4, 2020, https://www.nytimes.
    com/2020/05/04/us/coronavirus-live-updates.html

24 Colarossi, Natalie. "10 times Trump has lashed out at reporters."
    Business Insider, April 20, 2020, https://www.businessinsider.com/
    trump-lashes-out-at-reporters-during-coronavirus-press-brief-
    ings-2020-4

25 Wamsley, Laurel. "Rick Bright, Former Top Vaccine Scientist, Files
    Whistleblower Complaint." NPR, May 5, 2020, https://www.npr.

org/sections/coronavirus-live-updates/2020/05/05/850960344/
rick-bright-former-top-vaccine-scientist-files-whistleblower-
complaint

26 Wittes, Benjamin. "Why Is Trump's Inspector General Purge Not
a National Scandal?" Lawfare, April 8, 2020, https://www.lawfare-
blog.com/why-trumps-inspector-general-purge-not-national-scandal

27 Donnelly, John M. "Trump's pick for Pentagon
watchdog prompts questions." Roll Call, April
20, 2020, https://www.rollcall.com/2020/04/20/
trumps-pick-for-pentagon-watchdog-prompts-questions/

28 The White House. Kayleigh McEnany Press Conference Transcript.
May 6, 2020, https://www.rev.com/blog/transcripts/white-house-
press-secretary-kayleigh-mcenany-briefing-transcript-press-confer-
ence-may-6

Chapter Four

1 Brunk, Doug. "Remdesivir under study as treatment for novel
coronavirus." MDEdge, February 7, 2020, https://www.mdedge.
com/internalmedicine/article/216929/coronavirus-updates/
remdesivir-under-study-treatment-novel

2 Payne, Melanie. "Fact check: Did Florida county commissioner
propose a blow dryer cure for coronavirus?" USA Today, March
24, 2020.

3 Rana, S.V. et al. "Garlic hepatotoxicity: safe dose of garlic."
PubMed.gov, March 27, 2006, https://www.ncbi.nlm.nih.gov/
pubmed/16910057

4 Satariaino, Adam and Davey, Alba. "Burning Cell Towers, Out of
Baseless Fear They Spread the Virus." The New York Times, April
10, 2020, https://www.nytimes.com/2020/04/10/technology/
coronavirus-5g-uk.html

5 Eastburn, Kathryn. "Myths, misinformation about COVID-19
spread more quickly than the virus." The Daily News, Galveston
County, Texas, March 25,2020, https://www.galvnews.com/news/
free/article_d09f0fb1-0ca3-5447-9695-a28385f81eb6.html

6   Jamie P. "New COVID-19 Theory: Does Drinking Breast Milk Helpful vs Coronavirus?" Tech Times, April 14, 2020, https://www.techtimes.com/articles/248818/20200414/new-covid-19-theory-does-drinking-breastmilk-helpful-vs-coronavirus.htm

7   Gault, Matthew. "Iran's Fake Coronavirus Detector Is the Same as a Fake 'Bomb Detector.'" Vice.com, April 20, 2020, https://www.vice.com/en_us/article/k7edkx/irans-fake-coronavirus-detector-is-the-same-as-a-fake-bomb-detector

8   AgenceFrance-Presse. "Iran Guards Chief Vows 'Decisive Response' To US Gulf Threat." NDTV.com, April 23, 2020, https://www.ndtv.com/world-news/iran-guards-chief-major-general-hossein-salami-vows-decisive-response-to-us-gulf-threat-2217016

9   Kolata, Gina. "Is Ibuprofen Really Risky for Coronavirus Patients?" The New York Times, March 17, 2020, https://www.nytimes.com/2020/03/17/health/coronavirus-ibuprofen.html

10 Kolata, Gina. "Is Ibuprofen Really Risky for Coronavirus Patients?"

11 Reality Check Team. "Coronavirus: The fake health advice you should ignore." BBC News, March 8, 2020, https://www.bbc.com/news/world-51735367

12 Harvard Medical School. "Silver supplement warnings." Harvard Health Publishing, August 2007, https://www.health.harvard.edu/press_releases/silver-supplement-warnings

13 Smith, Michael W. "Can gargling with salt water or vinegar eliminate coronavirus?" WebMD.com, April 15, 2020, https://www.webmd.com/lung/qa/can-gargling-with-salt-water-or-vinegar-eliminate-coronavirus

14 Mitroff, Sarah. "8 coronavirus health myths, fact checked." C/NET, April 17, 2020, https://www.cnet.com/news/sensor-detects-coronavirus-covid-19-heart-problems/

15 Mitroff, Sarah. "8 coronavirus health myths, fact checked."

16 Buzz, "Should You Stop Having Ice-cream to Prevent Covid-19? This is What the Govt and WHO Say." News 18, April 30, 2020,

https://www.news18.com/news/buzz/should-you-stop-hav-ing-ice-cream-to-prevent-covid-19-this-is-what-the-govt-and-who-say-2599899.html

17 Goist, Robin. "No, you can't test for coronavirus by holding your breath or stop it by drinking water: Debunking COVID-19 myths." Cleveland.com, March 18,2020, https://www.cleveland.com/coronavirus/2020/03/no-you-cant-test-for-coronavirus-by-hold-ing-your-breath-or-stop-it-by-drinking-water-debunking-covid-19-myths.html

18 Parker-Pope, Tara. "Mixing Your Own Hand Sanitizer?" The New York Times, April 3, 2020, https://www.nytimes.com/article/coro-navirus-hand-sanitizer-home-made-diy.html

19 "Coronavirus myths explored." Medical News Today, May 7, 2020, https://www.medicalnewstoday.com/articles/coronavirus-myths-explored#What-should-we-do?

20 Scott, Mark. "It's Overwhelming: ON the frontline to combat coronavirus 'fake news.'" Politico, April 16, 2020, https://www.politico.eu/article/coronavirus-fake-news-fact-checkers-google-facebook-germany-spain-bosnia-brazil-united-states/

21 Wing, Daryl. "Coronavirus myths you need to ignore." Rentokil, April 28, 2020, https://www.rentokil.com/blog/coronavi-rus-myths/#.XsFaxr8rw6Y

22 Poynter Resources. "Fighting the infodemic: The #CoronaVirusFacts Alliance." Poynter, February 2, 2020, https://www.poynter.org/coronavirusfactsalliance/

23 Tompkins, Al. "Some restaurants have started tacking a COVID-19 surcharge onto customers' bills." Poynter, May 14, 2020, https://www.poynter.org/reporting-editing/2020/some-restaurants-have-started-tacking-a-covid-19-surcharge-onto-customers-bills/

24 Wong, Julia Carrie. "Tech giants struggle to stem 'info-demic' of false coronavirus claims." The Guardian, April 10, 2020, https://www.theguardian.com/world/2020/apr/10/tech-giants-struggle-stem-infodemic-false-coronavirus-claims

25　Linge, Mary Kay. "White House promises 27M coronavirus test kits by end of March." Fox News, March
22, 2020, https://www.foxnews.com/health/
white-house-promises-27m-coronavirus-test-kits-by-end-of-march

26　Bronstein, Scott et al. "Here's why the US is behind in coronavirus
testing." CNN, March 21, 2020, https://www.cnn.com/world/live-
news/coronavirus-outbreak-03-21-20-intl-hnk/h_78c4316624641
12a27434663a0860cdc

27　Forgey, Quint and Choi, Matthew. "Trump downplays need
for ventilators as New York begs to differ." Politico, March
27, 2020, https://www.politico.com/news/2020/03/26/
trump-ventilators-coronavirus-151311

28　MSN Lifestyle. "Meet the man who tracks the Fox-Trump feedback loop." MSN, January 19, 2020,https://www.msn.com/en-us/
tv/video/meet-the-man-who-tracks-the-fox-trump-feedback-loop/
vp-BBZ7EQn

29　Gertz, Mathew. "I've Studied the Trump-Fox Feedback Loop
for Months. It's Crazier Than You Think." Politico, January 5,
2020, https://www.politico.com/magazine/story/2018/01/05/
trump-media-feedback-loop-216248

30　Gertz, Mathew. "I've Studied the Trump-Fox Feedback Loop for
Months. It's Crazier Than You Think."

31　Ecarma, Caleb. "Fox News Goes Radio Silent on
Trump's Coronavirus Miracle Drug." Vanity Fair, April
22, 2020, https://www.vanityfair.com/news/2020/04/
fox-news-silent-trump-coronavirus-drug-hydroxychloroquine

32　Garcia, Victor. "Tucker Carlson blasts Trump critics as 'reac-
tive children' for dismissing hydroxychloroquine." Fox
News, March 25, 2020, https://www.foxnews.com/media/
tucker-carlson-blasts-trump-critics-hydroxychloroquine

33　Hickock, Kimberly. "Husband and wife poison themselves trying
to self-medicate with chloroquine." LiveScience, March 24, 2020,
https://www.livescience.com/coronavirus-chloroquine-self-medica-
tion-kills-man.html

34 Hickock, Kimberly. "Husband and wife poison themselves trying to self-medicate with chloroquine."

35 Infectious Diseases Editors. "Coronavirus Disease 2019: Myth vs. Fact." Johns Hopkins Medicine, April 27, 2020, https://www.hopkinsmedicine.org/health/conditions-and-diseases/coronavirus/2019-novel-coronavirus-myth-versus-fact

36 Yeo, Amanda. "Do not inject yourself with bleach to cure coronavirus, holy crap." Mashable, April 24, 2020, https://mashable.com/article/inject-bleach-donald-trump-coronavirus-drink-disinfectant-ultraviolet-light/

37 Johnson, Ted. "It Is A Matter Of Life And Death": Donald Trump's Disinfectant Comments Still Trigger Alarm Even After He Claimed He Was Being Sarcastic." Deadline, April 24, 2020, https://deadline.com/2020/04/coronavirus-donald-trump-disinfectant-sanjay-gupta-1202917480/

38 Glater, Robert, MD. "Calls To Poison Centers Spike After The President's Comments About Using Disinfectants To Treat Coronavirus." Forbes, April 25, 2020, https://www.forbes.com/sites/robertglatter/2020/04/25/calls-to-poison-centers-spike--after-the-presidents-comments-about-using-disinfectants-to-treat-coronavirus/#54f5c1711157

39 Glater, Robert, MD. "Calls To Poison Centers Spike After The President's Comments About Using Disinfectants To Treat Coronavirus."

40 Editors. "Hand Sanitizer." American Association of Poison Control Centers. April 30, 2020, https://aapcc.org/track/hand-sanitizer

41 Editors. "NCI Dictionary of Cancer Terms." NIH National Cancer Institute. https://www.cancer.gov/publications/dictionaries/cancer-terms/def/797584

42 Editors. "Shutsung Liao, 1931-2014." UChicagoNews, July 28,2014, https://news.uchicago.edu/story/shutsung-liao-biochemist/

43 King, Stephen. The Stand: <u>The Complete and Uncut Edition.</u> New York: Doubleday, 1978, rev. 1990, p. 114.

44 King, Carole and Goffin, Gerry. "Wasn't Born to Follow." From <u>The Notorious Byrd Brothers</u>. Los Angeles: Columbia Studios, 1968.

Chapter Five

1 Center for Disease Control and Prevention. "Testing Data in the U.S." May 29, 2020, https://www.cdc.gov/coronavirus/2019-ncov/cases-updates/testing-in-us.html

2 S.R. Hadden to Ellie Arroway in <u>Contact</u>.

3 Rabinovitch-Fox, Einav. "The fashionable history of social distancing." <u>The Conversation</u>, March 26, 2020, https://theconversation.com/the-fashionable-history-of-social-distancing-134464

4 Dawsey, Josh. "Trump derides protections for immigrants from 'shithole' countries." <u>The Washington Post</u>, January 12, 2018, https://www.washingtonpost.com/politics/trump-attacks-protections-for-immigrants-from-shithole-countries-in-oval-office-meeting/2018/01/11/bfc0725c-f711-11e7-91af-31ac729add94_story.html

5 Levitan, Richard MD. "The Infection That's Silently Killing Coronavirus Patients." <u>The New York Times</u>, April 20, 202, https://www.nytimes.com/2020/04/20/opinion/sunday/coronavirus-testing-pneumonia.html

6 Dan O'Herlihy to Russell Hardie in Sidney Lumet's 1964 film <u>Fail-Safe</u>.

7 Rauf, Don and Laube, Justin, MD. "Do Steroid Meds Up My Risk of COVID-19 or Getting Sicker From It?" <u>Everyday Health</u>, April 21, 2020, https://www.everydayhealth.com/coronavirus/do-steroid-meds-up-my-risk-of-covid-19-or-getting-sicker-from-it/

8 JCME Editors. "Individuals taking class of steroid medications at high risk for COVID-19 " <u>Endocrine Society</u>, March 31,2020, https://www.endocrine.org/news-and-advocacy/news-room/2020/

individuals-taking-class-of-steroid-medications-at-high-risk-
for-covid

9   Archibald, Ben. "BREACH BUMS Coronavirus Scotland:
    Fuming Ayrshire pensioners claim nudist influx breaking
    lockdown at local beach." The Scottish Sun, May 15,
    2020, https://www.thescottishsun.co.uk/news/5600552/
    coronavirus-scotland-ayrshire-pensioner-nudist-lockdown-beach/

Chapter Six

1   "Wuhan's 'wet markets' are back in business." ABC News,
    April 17, 2020, https://abcnews.go.com/International/
    wuhans-called-wet-markets-back-business/story?id=70119116

2   Bump, Philip. How Trump's rhetoric on testing in the U.S. com-
    pared with what was — or wasn't — being done." The Washington
    Post, March 31, 2020, https://www.washingtonpost.com/poli-
    tics/2020/03/31/how-trumps-rhetoric-testing-us-compared-with-
    what-was-or-wasnt-being-done/

3   Eban, Katherine. "'Really Want to Flood NY and
    NJ': Internal Documents Reveal Team Trump's
    Chloroquine Master Plan." Vanity Fair, April 24,
    2020, https://www.vanityfair.com/news/2020/04/
    internal-documents-reveal-team-trumps-chloroquine-master-plan

4   "Opening Up America Again." https://www.whitehouse.gov/
    openingamerica/

5   Maxouris, Christine et al. "As of Wednesday, every state will be
    somewhere along the road toward a full reopening." CNN, May
    19, 2020, https://www.cnn.com/2020/05/19/health/us-coronavi-
    rus-tuesday/index.html

6   Hansen, Claire. "Projected U.S. Coronavirus Deaths Jump
    as States Reopen." U.S. News, May 12, 2020, https://www.
    usnews.com/news/national-news/articles/2020-05-12/
    projected-us-coronavirus-deaths-jump-as-states-reopen

7   Buettner, Dan. "COVID-19: Straight Answers from Top
    Epidemiologist Who Predicted the Pandemic." Blue Zones, June 9,

2020, https://www.bluezones.com/2020/06/covid-19-straight-answers-from-top-epidemiologist-who-predicted-the-pandemic/

8   Song lyrics from the end credits of the 1970 Robert Rush film Getting Straight.

9   Blue Cheer. "Second Time Around." <u>Vincebus Eruptum</u>. New York: Polygram Records, 1967.

10 Thompson, Hunter S. <u>Generation of Swine: Gonzo Papers, Vol. 2</u>. New York: Summit Books, 1988, p. 51.

11 Flogging Molly. "The Worst Day Since Yesterday." <u>Swagger</u>. Dublin: SideOneDummy, 2000.

12 Ross, George H. <u>Trump Strategies for Real Estate</u>. Hoboken: John Wiley & Sons, 2005, p. 56.

13 Gerry Lane, in a voiceover at the end of <u>World War Z</u>.

CPSIA information can be obtained
at www.ICGtesting.com
Printed in the USA
LVHW082351181221
706606LV00009B/29/J